ENVY IN EVERYDAY LIFE

ENVY IN EVERYDAY LIFE

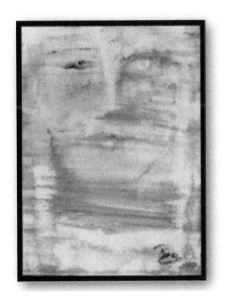

Patricia Polledri

2016

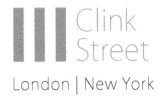

Clink
Street

London | New York

Published by Clink Street Publishing 2016

Copyright © 2016

First edition.

ISBN 978-1-911110-26-2 paperback
ISBN 978-1-911110-27-9 ebook

Virtually all people, including the most primitive, have found it necessary to define the state of mind of a person who cannot bear someone else's being something, having a skill, possessing something or enjoying a reputation which he himself lacks, and who will therefore rejoice should the other lose his asset, although the loss will not mean his own gain.

HELMUT SCHOECK, *ENVY: A THEORY OF SOCIAL BEHAVIOUR*, 1987

CONTENTS

ACKNOWLEDGEMENTS

THE EARLY DEVELOPMENT of my ideas about the psychopathology of envy was greatly facilitated by the insightful comments and support of several inspirational teachers, mentors and supervisors who range across the whole spectrum of the human sciences.

One of my deepest debts, and certainly the most specific one, is to the many men and women I have treated in my twenty-five years of clinical experience who were detained in various prisons, special hospitals and psychiatric clinics in the United Kingdom. Without their help this book absolutely could not have been written. Where I have quoted, paraphrased or summarized what they have said, I have not used their names or any identifying information in order to protect their privacy.

AUTHOR'S NOTE

DESPITE THEIR IDENTITY in sound and in ultimate etymology, 'fantasy' and 'phantasy' tend to be apprehended as separate words, the predominant sense of fantasy, according to the British psychiatrist and psychoanalyst Charles Rycroft, being 'caprice, whim, fanciful invention', while phantasy is 'imagination, visionary notion'. Since the psychoanalytical concept is more akin to imagination than whimsy, I have used the spelling 'phantasy' throughout.

Rather than use the cumbersome he/she throughout, I have used the masculine pronoun in general contexts.

INTRODUCTION: THE PSYCHOANALYTIC BACKGROUND

Envy is a mushroom of an emotion. It grows in darkness.

LAURIE BECKELMAN, *ENVY*, 1995

A MAJOR FACTOR for me in writing this book is that the concept of envy has been actively banished from conscious thought, as well as from the social sciences and philosophy, since the turn of the century, possibly because it is so unpleasant to admit to. Yet envy plays an important role in all societies. There are crimes of envy, politics based on envy, institutions designed to regulate envy and powerful reasons to avoid being envied by others. Failing to develop a thesis that allows us to understand envy can cost us dear, so the time has come to give envy its due.

An in-depth study of one of the mind's most misunderstood states, this book is intended to be a seedbed of information about the subject. It is important to emphasize the ways in which we come across envy in everyday life, sometimes without even being aware of it. We need to know more about how to describe it, what causes it and how we can identify it should we or a loved one become the target of an envious attack.

There are, of course, positive and stimulating encounters that encourage us to give our best in everyday life; but there are others that can undermine and ultimately destroy us. When envy is in action, it is akin to emotional abuse. One individual can succeed in destroying another by a process that culminates in a virtual murder of the soul.

Historically, most of the academic literature on the subject of envy derives from the work of the psychoanalyst Melanie Klein (1882–1960) and her followers, who have written extensively about it since the late 1940s. In fact, the title of this book is taken from a 1986 paper by the psychoanalyst Betty Joseph, a contemporary of Klein.

Klein claimed that we are all born envious, it is constitutional, and that, among other things, babies attack their mother's breast, by biting it, out of envy at her capacity to supply milk in abundance.[1] Attempts to question or challenge that theory have been rejected or devalued by the Kleinians and so, for them, it holds true to this day in the field of psychoanalysis.

In this book I intend to unpack the dense theoretical jargon and to provide readers with a more accessible, modern approach, written in plain English, towards a subject that should be of interest to everyone.

I first wrote about envy in an attempt to update the literature in *Envy is Not Innate: A New Model of Thinking* (2012). This was a textbook for those working in the field of forensic psychiatry and was the result of many years' clinical and theoretical research. The book was well received by academics, but the main comment I had from family and friends was that it was too difficult to read for even the intelligent layperson. As a response to this very valuable feedback, I have now written what I hope is a clearer, less academic version that will be easier to read for those who are interested in this perplexing, fascinating and yet ultimately destructive phenomenon.

In terms of understanding envy, I believe that if a child's self-esteem is undernourished during its developmental years, the sense of self becomes weak, which results in a lasting narcissistic hunger that manifests itself in envy of others who have had, to use Donald Winnicott's term, a 'good enough' – that is, a more supportive – childhood. This, in turn, easily activates destructiveness towards those others.

I will demonstrate how we come across envy on a daily basis, whether we recognize it or not. Envy is so unpleasant, negative and corrosive that often we would rather not think about it or devote any energy to it. In my experience, envy is harmful to the recipient precisely because it is never out in the open, as I will go on to describe. I have had twenty-five years' clinical experience with a wide range of individuals in which to develop my understanding of envy. Therefore I know that it is crucial for our well-being to be able to identify when we are on the receiving end of a destructive envious attack, be it from a friend, a lover, a work colleague, a sibling, a parent or any other individual with whom we are in contact on a regular basis – or even when it is a one-off attack.

In order to examine envy in all its different guises, I will break it down into its various forms. Having first explained the difference between jealousy and envy, I will then consider what is meant by the word Schadenfreude, how shame is a component of envy, how we can be envious of ourselves, how envy is an underlying factor in perverse behaviour, what is meant by womb envy, how envious individuals are totally lacking in empathy, why narcissist traits are always linked to envious individuals and why I consider envy to be emotional abuse. I will follow this by considering how envy exists in academic institutions and in the workplace, explaining why I think that most envious individuals can be seen as having a mental disorder but not a psychiatric illness. I will introduce the term 'forensic psychotherapy' in relation to a discussion of the trial of the South African athlete Oscar Pistorius, demonstrating how his behaviour was an example of what Kant called 'envy in action' and, in conclusion, explain why I believe, unlike Melanie Klein and her followers, that envy is not innate – that is, that we are not all born envious.

Everything I write here is to help you to understand envy and to protect yourself when you see it in others. Envy was identified as one of humanity's greatest problems long before we had heard of psychoanalysis and appears in the list of the seven deadly sins. Indeed, in 'The Parson's Tale' Chaucer refers to it as the worst sin there is. From ancient times, philosophers have devoted their attentions to the subject and literature is full of examples.

According to Klein, envy is directed at all virtue and all goodness; the envious man sickens at the sight of enjoyment, happy only in the misery of others.[2] I recently had a conversation with someone who was describing his reaction to the news that his wife had not got the high-powered job she had just applied for. He told me how in the past:

> *I found myself enjoying it when things went badly for her at work ... on the occasions she texted me saying something had gone wrong I found myself looking forward to the evening, when I could pretend to comfort her ... I also started making excuses not to attend occasions when she would be having drinks to celebrate getting a new contract ... If I did go, the taxi ride home would end in an argument as my wife struggled to understand why I had been so stand-offish ... and when she would sometimes come home from work, eyes shining, after being praised by her boss, I'd think ... I wonder how long it will take me to wipe that smile off your face ...*

This young man then embarked on numerous affairs during their marriage, which is an indication that infidelity can also be based on envy of one's partner, leaving the other in utter despair.

Although I will provide examples such as these throughout the book to illustrate the main thrust of my argument, that envy is never out in the open, it will soon become clear that feelings of envy and resentment are always triggered by another's success. I can see that it is very tempting to play down one's own successes to appease an insecure partner, but this is not the answer. The more one survives an envious attack, the more enviable one becomes to the other and the attacks increase.

We might envy someone's personality, success, possessions, sense of humour, talent, beauty, intelligence or popularity. Sometimes envy of what we perceive someone else to have can hurt so badly that we want to destroy it. We have grown up knowing from a very early age that envy is 'bad'. In fairy tales, envious people are depicted as ugly and mean-spirited. What's more, they don't just feel envy, they act on it: the impulse becomes so unbearable that action against the envied other is the only relief, however temporary it might be. But in fairy tales bad things tend to happen to envious people. After all, Cinderella's stepsisters aren't the ones who get the prince in the end. And when the evil stepmother tries to kill Snow White, whose beauty and virtue she envies, it is she, not Snow

White, who dies a hideous death. Memorable fables like these are not the only age-old warnings against envy.

Envy can consume the envier, who lives on a treadmill. It has been described thus: when your gain is my pain and your pain is my gain. Envy can poison the mind of the envier and it is this malevolence that we are warned against. Even if envy is denied or ignored, it will still continue to fester, because, as Laurie Beckelman noted, it is a mushroom of an emotion that flourishes in dark places.

PART I: DESCRIBING ENVY

CHAPTER 1

JEALOUSY AND ENVY

O, beware, my lord, of jealousy;
It is the green-eyed monster which doth mock
The meat it feeds on ...

OTHELLO, ACT III, SCENE 3

IN DISCUSSIONS WITH people about what they understand by envy, I have been struck by how many times the word 'jealousy' is used instead of 'envy'. It is important to distinguish between them, although the two are often closely linked and overlap.

Basically, envy occurs when one person feels they lack what another person has and wishes that the other person did not have it. The first person does not want what the other person has for himself, but spoils it so that the other person cannot enjoy having it. Jealousy, on the other hand, occurs when a person either fears losing or has already lost an important relationship with another person to a rival. Jealousy may be felt in many different ways, but typically it includes fear of loss, anger over betrayal and insecurity. Jealousy implies that there is someone or something we want to possess.

Jealousy occurs in the context of relationships. With jealousy, three people need to be involved: the couple and the outsider who is jealous of them and wishes to spoil their relationship. We all carry the 'jealousy gene'; we are born with it and it is, unlike envy, innate. Our parents were united in their sexual relationship for us to be conceived. We are therefore on the outside of that triangular relationship from the day we are born.

In his 1988 book *The Tyranny of Malice*, the psychoanalyst and psychiatrist Joseph Berke states that, in adulthood, love scorned is a central theme in the loss of a beloved to another. When this happens, or even if there is a threat of it happening, jealous passions soon erupt. Alternatively, the jealous person may be the outsider, an excluded third party full of desire who comes between two others so that a new loving relationship can begin.

To further highlight the difference between jealousy and envy, I will quote from the author and journalist Jilly Cooper, someone who skilfully wrote any number of successful racy and romantic novels. In her own life, though, she describes this painful triangular situation in her reaction of jealous possessiveness when she thinks her husband is with another woman:

> *About once a year something triggers off a really bad attack of jealousy, and I turn into a raving maniac, all perspective blotted out. 'He's late home from work,' I reason. 'He must be with another woman.' Or he's early. 'He must be feeling guilty about having a boozy lunch with her.' And so on and so on, lashing myself with misery. Once the octopus jealousy gets me in its stranglehold, it is almost impossible to wriggle free.*[1]

This is the difference between jealousy, involving a triangular relationship, and envy, which involves only one other person. Here, love is the primary issue, not hate. However, jealous anger and hatred can be quite as cruel, malicious and spiteful as envy. What differs is the focus – love lost; the direction of the anger – towards the rival; and the possibility of a resolution – love regained and retained.

Jealousy is also popularly associated with sexual jealousy, the subject of countless films, plays and books. The themes are always irrationality, infidelity, passion and possessiveness. These issues relating to jealousy arise from relationships, whether sexually orientated or not, to the exclusion of someone else. Jealousy is also group-orientated, as it involves a threesome.

By contrast, envy is a more primitive emotional state and is not concerned with relationships as such. It needs only one other person. Definitions of envy emphasize feelings of hostility, spite and ill-will. Envy is a directed emotion: without a victim, it cannot occur. It is also called envy when a person withholds something from someone else out of spite and the other person is not aware of it. Here I can give an example of something that happened to me when it was my turn to host an annual gathering of work colleagues. I was preparing a dinner for eight people and I asked a colleague to let the others know the date and time. I assumed she had done so, but it 'slipped her mind'. I was left with a table full of food and no guests, feeling a complete fool. When I called her, assuming I had got the date wrong, she said, 'Oh no, you poor thing. I was waiting for you to reconfirm the date.'

I had been reduced from a qualified, competent forensic specialist to a "poor thing". I had innocently trusted her to pass on the details. This is an example of inaction, withholding something by 'forgetting' to pass on important information. It is always deliberate, but it is never out in the open.

At the time, I had the opportunity to spend some time in discussion with Joseph Berke (whose work I will quote from regularly throughout this book) and he gave me valuable insights into the many unresolved questions I had about envy. Berke describes envy as a state of exquisite tension, torment and ill-will provoked by an overwhelming sense of inferiority, impotence and worthlessness. He believes it begins in the eye of the beholder and is so painful to the mind that the envious person will go to almost any lengths to diminish, if not destroy, whatever and whoever may have aroused it.[2]

Begrudging and a sense of injustice are characteristic of envious people, who take pleasure in depriving others of what they have or could have, without deriving any sort of advantage themselves. Such individuals go to great lengths to inflict harm and unhappiness. Envious destructiveness is deliberate. The envious person denies goodwill or love towards the recipient of his anger. What he wants is to remove the bilious anger and bitter vindictiveness from within himself, to get rid of it and put it elsewhere. Since he blames what he envies for how he feels, he sets out to make it feel or appear bad. Any relief is temporary, because the source of his torment is not in what he envies but in himself. I will describe this in more detail in the chapter on Oscar Pistorius, who shot and killed his girlfriend, Reeva Steenkamp, in 2013, claiming that he thought she was an intruder.

A very penetrating and useful distinction between envy and jealousy drawn by the American psychoanalyst Harry Stack Sullivan fifty years ago, based upon the two- or three-person model, neatly summarizes matters:

> *Let me discriminate my meaning of the terms jealousy and envy, which are often tossed around as synonyms. There is a fundamental difference in the felt components of envy and jealousy, and there also is a fundamental difference in the interpersonal situations in which these processes occur, for envy occurs in a two-person relationship, while jealousy always appears in a relationship involving a group of three. I define envy, which is more widespread in our social organization than jealousy, as pertaining to personal attachments or attributes. Envy is an activity in which one contemplates the unfortunate results of someone else's having something that one does not have.*
>
> *Jealousy, on the other hand, never concerns a two-person situation. It is invariably a very complex, painful process involving a group of three persons, one or more of whom may be absolutely fantasized. Jealousy is much more poignant and devastating than envy; in contrast with envy, it does not concern itself with an attribute or an attachment, but, rather, involves a great complex field of interpersonal relations. [3]*

Sullivan rightly recognizes the relationship between self-pity and envy. Although he in no way sees envy itself as self-pity, the latter may sometimes take its place. Self-pity arises in diverse situations, when a person who already has a low opinion of himself gets into difficulties. It eliminates envious comparison with others that might otherwise endanger self-esteem.

Both envy and jealousy are of great importance in social life and can be powerful motivators of behaviour.

CHAPTER 2

ENVY IS AS OLD AS MANKIND

*Socrates: Did we not say that pleasure
in the misfortune of
friends was caused by envy?*

PLATO, *PHILEBUS*

I DON'T BELIEVE we are all born envious or that envy is innate or constitutional. I see it rather as a disturbance in attachment, way back in in-
fancy and childhood, to our primary carer/mother, which can be part
and parcel of normal development that has gone wrong. This unhappy
experience affects an individual's self-esteem and confidence, which can
lead on to the development of a malignant pathology. Envy then becomes the angry feeling that someone else possesses and is enjoying
something desirable, the envious impulse being to take it away and spoil
it. This is what I have learned at the coalface, having worked for many
years with individuals in the field of forensic psychiatry and psychotherapy. But this is also what can be seen from the works of any number of
philosophers and writers, for envy has been around a very long time.

ENVY IN THE BIBLE: SIBLING RIVALRY

Sibling rivalry is a term used to describe the very natural and normal envy
between brothers and sisters. It is so typical that we can safely say it is a
common feature of family life. Siblings compete for their parents' atten-

tion. Of course, some parents really do favour one child over another. The biblical stories of Cain and Abel and Esau and Jacob are good examples of disappointed love, parental rejection and subsequent hatred displaced on to a brother. And some children, with or without siblings, truly are deprived. Their parents or other carers may be unable to meet their needs for any number of reasons, including illness, alcoholism, drug abuse or stress due to job loss, divorce, poverty or family difficulties. But the envy in sibling rivalry experienced in early relationships within the family carries over into later life. Symptoms of this unresolved early envy are likely to be:

- a sense of injustice and being deprived of something we feel we deserve
- comparing ourselves with someone who has what we want
- feeling powerless to change a situation and so setting out to destroy it
- believing we can't have what we want as long as the other person has it

The first urge of envy is not 'I, too, must have what he has' but 'I want him not to have what he has, because it makes me feel less than I am.'

I remember a young man I met many years ago who had worked hard throughout the Christmas holidays to finish his dissertation for his degree. His older brother had referred to him as 'the golden boy' throughout his life, perceiving him to be cleverer. The older brother took the precious piece of work and promised to post it to the university for his younger brother, who had developed a very serious eye infection and could not do so himself. The dissertation never arrived at the university to meet the deadline. It was mysteriously 'lost in the post'. This was before the days of computers, so there was no other copy for him to send as a replacement. Of course, his envious brother 'forgot' to send it by registered post!

ENVY IN SHAKESPEARE: THE MOOR OF VENICE

Shakespeare's greatness is in large part due to the fact that he was an incredibly perceptive analyst of the human psyche. The characters in his masterpiece *Othello* embody envy and jealousy. In this dramatic story, Iago is driven by his relentless envy of Othello, the Moor, and Othello's new wife, Desdemona. They have married in secret as Desdemona's father would not have given his permission for this mixed-race marriage, though theirs is a relationship built on mutual love and respect. Iago has other grievances too: the promotion of Cassio over him to become Othello's lieutenant, and his resentment at no longer receiving money from Rodrigo, who had been paying him to be the go-between for himself and Desdemona, a situation now patently untenable. He also has a paranoid suspicion that Othello has had an affair with his own wife, Emilia. Rather than taking steps to find out whether this is true or false, he determines to:

> *... put the Moor*
> *At least into a jealousy so strong*
> *That judgement cannot cure ...*

In my experience, all envious individuals are paranoid. Iago projects his own jealousy, lack of judgement and inability to test reality on to Othello and seems to have no interest in the truth. He is exploiting his own and Othello's feelings for the purpose of manipulation, to bring about Othello's downfall.

One of the qualities most envied in life generally by the envious is peace of mind. Other enviable qualities are goodness and innocence ... the absence of envy in the other. Iago cannot bear these qualities in either Othello or Desdemona and his plans are based on the ruin of Desdemona's goodness and innocence. Iago is an expert in manipulative envy: he knows exactly how to ensnare his enemy and he does it remorselessly. He supplants his knowledge of the sexuality of the couple and the thought of their progeny with his own monstrous conception. When Othello eventually destroys Desdemona, the story shows the power of manipulative envy, the aim of which is devastation. Iago knows he will gain nothing from his plans except the triumph of destruction, which is vintage envy!

Nowadays, envy is just as prevalent as it was in Shakespeare's time, but people are less straightforward about it, as the emotional meaning and motivation of the term tend to be clouded.

ENVY AND THE PHILOSOPHERS

The Germans have a lovely word that describes how we often cope with envy: Schadenfreude. Literally 'harm-joy', it is the gloating sense of pleasure we get when we see another person suffer. We particularly seek Schadenfreude when thinking about people we envy – an emotion that the press tap into when they publish stories about the downfall of the rich and famous. The opposite of Schadenfreude is *mudita,* a Hindu word meaning delight in the good fortune of others.

A particularly dangerous aspect of envy is not envy itself but the denial of it, as the envious impulse cannot be modified by loving, reparative wishes. The envier will use powerful projective processes – that is, the very mechanism of envy – to dissociate from a major part of himself ... his own destructiveness.

Among the seven deadly sins, envy is the one that has no obvious pleasure attached to it. Immanuel Kant, in his late work *The Metaphysics of Morals* (1797), discusses envy, which he regards as belonging to the 'abhorrent family of ingratitude and Schadenfreude'. This he refers to as 'The vice of human hate that is the complete opposite of human love. [It is a hate that is] not open and violent, but secret and disguised, so that baseness is added to neglect of one's duty to one's neighbour, and thus one's duty to oneself also suffers.' Kant gives full expression to the philosophical doctrine and ethic of values, according to which envy is the very antithesis of virtue, the denial of humanity.[1]

Arthur Schopenhauer recalls that of all animals man alone torments his own kind for entertainment. This leads him on to an analysis of envy: 'The worst trait in human nature, however, is *Schadenfreude,* for it is closely related to cruelty … generally … appearing where compassion should find a place … In another sense, envy is opposed to compassion, since it stems from an opposite cause.'

Envy, Schopenhauer believes, has two favourite methods: to praise what is bad or, alternatively, to remain silent about what is good. Among his remarks, he includes a quotation from an article in *The Times* of 9 October 1858, a passage which gives 'the most adorned and strongest expression' to the fact that envy 'is irreconcilable in regard to personal advantages':

There is no vice, of which a man can be guilty, no meanness, no shabbiness, no unkindness, which excites so much indignation among his contemporaries, friends and neighbours, as his success. This is the one unpardonable crime, which reason cannot defend, nor humility mitigate.
'When heaven with such parts has blest him,
Have I not reason to detest him?'
is a genuine and natural expression of the vulgar human mind. The man who writes as we cannot write, who speaks as we cannot speak, labours as we cannot labour, thrives as we cannot thrive, has accumulated on his own person all the offences of which man can be guilty. Down with him! Why cumbereth he the ground? … [2]

According to Søren Kierkegaard, mistrust belongs to the same genus as envy, as do Schadenfreude and baseness. He writes:

And there is envy; it is quick to abandon a man, and yet it does not abandon him as it were by letting him go, no, it hastens to assist his fall. And this being once assured, envy will hasten to his dark corner whence he will summon his even more hideous cousin, malicious glee, that they may rejoice together – at their own cost. [3]

Friedrich Nietzsche, like Kierkegaard and Schopenhauer, also recognized the function of envy in human society. The force of his observations must be attributed to countless experiences of being envied. His entire opus, from first to last, contains references to the problem of envy, but they are most abundant in his middle period, of which the central work is *Human, All Too Human* (1878). As a classical philologist, he was familiar with the Greek idea of the envy of the gods. He had, however, a tendency to idealize this and, like Kierkegaard, to underestimate the full import of envious manifestations in Athenian democracy. Nietzsche does not confuse the concepts jealousy and envy, as so many of his predecessors and successors have repeatedly done, but he does describe resentment beautifully in his *On the Genealogy of Morality* (1887):

> *All men of resentment are those physiologically distorted and worm-riddled persons, a whole quivering kingdom of burrowing revenge, indefatigable and insatiable in its outbursts against the happy, and equally so in disguises for revenge, in pretexts for revenge: when will they really reach their final, fondest, most sublime triumph of revenge? At that time, doubtless, when they succeed in pushing their own misery, indeed all misery there is, into the consciousness of the happy; so that the latter begin one day to be ashamed of their happiness, and perchance say to themselves when they meet, it is a shame to be happy!* There is too much misery![4]

Nietzsche examines resentment in many forms, and also its physiological manifestations, as a reactive and enduring mode of behaviour. But he regards envy as more comprehensive than jealousy.

PART II: ENVY IN ACTION

CHAPTER 3

SHAME AND ENVY

The bird of hope landed softly on my perch
With her sweet song she flirted, and enchanted me,
Then spread her coloured wings, as I pursued her,
Soaring high, and low,
We rested in the forest, where she dallied with another,
Then the black knight of jealousy,
riding roughshod in my heart,
Trampled her to death.
And I was ashamed.

QUOTED IN PHIL MOLLON, *SHAME AND JEALOUSY*, 2002

IT IS CLEAR to me that shame is always combined with envy – a view that Joseph Berke encouraged me to discuss in this book. Shame is a powerful inner tension experienced as an exquisitely painful sense of inferiority at variance with one's wished-for image of personal goodness. With shame, the quality and degree of emotional pain are comparable to those of envious tension, so much so that shameful tension is likely to be a variant of, as well as a contributor to, envy. If this is correct, then we would expect shame to be followed by murderous rage. In my clinical experience working in the field of forensic psychiatry and psychotherapy, this is generally the case.

The shamed person wants to hide away, to disappear, as the envier does at times, but also wants to attack and destroy the alleged source of

17

shame. With shame, as with envy, a tormenting tension leads to an angry outburst. But with shame it is the tension that most people recognize. They tend to overlook the subsequent response.[1]

So how does shame develop and how is it related to envy?

Shame develops very early on in life through an unreflecting look in the mother's eyes, well before the development of language.[2] Eye contact is one of the core means by which we communicate and build relationships, and is the key mechanism by which we develop attachments. Gaze avoidance or an inability to sustain eye contact is an important signal about the state of the relationship with or the emotional state of the individual involved.[3] This unreflecting look is then internalized by the infant as an experience, well before verbal shaming comments, depending on the tone of voice, which then reverberate throughout later life.

The child can experience a look in the mother's eyes, a look that lacks a reflective capacity, forcing an awareness of worthlessness on to the child's immature, fragile ego, perhaps due to the mother's own disturbance in attachment to *her* mother in childhood. The eyes of shame are a concrete, unsymbolized representation of a sensory experience of an uncontaining mother – a mother who cannot hold feeling, who has no empathy – leaving the child feeling what British psychoanalyst and pioneer of child development Donald Winnicott describes in his 1971 book *Playing and Reality* as 'not good enough'.[4] From this it is evident that the eye is the organ of shame par excellence.

Children cannot know who they are without reflective mirroring. Parents who are shut down emotionally cannot mirror or affirm their child's emotions. Our identity demands a significant other whose eyes see us pretty much as we see ourselves. Envy uses disguises to cover up the core issue, which is toxic shame. Because of its talent for disguise, envy takes forms that are impossible to recognize.[5]

It seems to me that the fixed face of the unresponsive mother is experienced by the infant as a reflection, but a distorting one, giving a false feedback of deadness. I am suggesting that during the first six months of life, it appears that the subsequent development of a sense of shame is linked to the role the eyes play for the infant in constructing the mother's presence and forming the psychological centre of their relationship.

The British psychotherapist Phil Mollon has written an interesting book about the subject, *Shame and Jealousy* (2002), in which he describes shame as being about a broken connection between one human being and others, a breach in the understanding, expectation and acceptance that are necessary for a sense of being a valued member of the human family. The cure for shame is the empathy provided by another.

During my time as a researcher of Munchausen Syndrome by Proxy, working with mothers who harmed or killed their children, typical comments I heard from an envious mother were, 'When I looked at my baby, I just couldn't bond with "it". There was something missing', and then, 'Of course I felt guilty, but I couldn't understand what all the fuss was about.' As this woman had had a very unhappy experience with her own drug-addicted mother as an infant, she repeatedly said, 'I didn't have a loving mother and I survived. What do you expect?' This was very common with those who had narcissistic mothers and those with mothers who had problems with alcohol and drug abuse. There was an underlying sense of shame, covered up by defensive behaviour, which in turn created a perversion of the maternal instinct.

On the other hand, I have also talked to mothers who have acknowledged that although they had a cold and unresponsive mother during their early years they were determined not to repeat the pattern. These mothers usually had a kind grandparent or other family members who were there for them.

Rage and violence may also, paradoxically, increase the feelings of shame that they were originally intended to provide protection from. I consulted James Gilligan, a prison psychiatrist in Boston, USA, with considerable experience of analysing violent men, about shame and its relation to envy. Envy is a reaction to deep-seated feelings of inadequacy about which the individual is tremendously ashamed. Violence hides a fundamental sense of shame, and it enables the perpetrators to hide their most vulnerable self. Violence serves as a smokescreen, a defence that hides the unacceptable 'unmanly' desire to be taken care of: a wish that, if granted, would make many a man feel that he was passive, dependent, infantile and weak – that is to say, 'not a man'.

Gilligan said that in his violent men, they would like nothing better than to be thought of as filled with 'aggressive instincts'. Nothing is more flattering to the shaky self-esteem of a man who fears he is 'really a wimp' than to be told, and to believe, that he is actually carrying within himself very dangerous instincts; it avoids having to contemplate the shameful thought that men need to be helped by each other, and even more shamefully by a woman! [6]

Finally, a certain number of individuals handle shame by attacking others through the 'human sport' of put-down, humiliation, ridicule, contempt, 'constructive criticism' and character assassination. These are the people in our everyday lives most of us find extremely dangerous, for no one can really avoid shame successfully and we live at risk of their envy. Those who must attack, rather than withdraw, make our common ground a hazardous place. [7]

CHAPTER 4

SELF-ENVY

A dog was once crossing a bridge over a river, and in his jaws was a piece of meat. When he saw his reflection in the water, he thought he saw another dog under the water with an equally large piece of meat. In his greed he leapt at the other dog, not realizing that he and it were one and the same, and lost both his meat and the meat he coveted.

AESOP, 'THE DOG AND HIS SHADOW'

HOW CAN ONE ENVY oneself for what one in fact has?

Self-envy arises as a result of an early traumatic experience in relating. It starts with the mother not being able to 'tune in' to her baby over the developmental years. There are many causes for this, including mental illness, depression or a failure in the mother to have bonded with her own mother. As our significant other, our mother, as carer, interacts with us during these dependent times, when we develop experiences of the mind, such as thoughts, emotions, perceptions and memories. If all goes well we become relatively sane individuals who are able, in turn, to form attachments to others in later life.

If healthy bonding has been denied to the developing child, an inner world is constructed which is divided into two parts. The emphasis of self-envy is then based on the relationship between those two internal parts of the self.

This does not mean that we cannot form relationships in the outside world. We can. It is the relationship between the two parts of ourselves, in our head or in our mind, that also effects what goes on in the relationships outside ourselves with others. This has a major influence on how we relate to our partners.

Clinically, I have found that self-envy also affects the relationship between therapist and patient. It is extremely difficult to identify, as I discovered over many years of trying to understand this behaviour in my consulting room. The experience left me so puzzled that I was curious about how the situation develops. The presenting problem is an overwhelming sense of negativity and depression that is always in the background. This is often described as a 'black hole', or 'my demons', or 'my other self', or 'my nasty twin'. This nasty other self behaves like a cynical internal observer trying to spoil the person's life.

This must not be confused with schizophrenia or hearing voices. It is a part of us that has a powerful authority and is given almost as much credence as our instinct, so we trust it. But it is a destructive part and should not be given any energy.

Self-envy can also be understood as the begrudging part of those children who resent their parents' capacity to reproduce and can be the bedrock of sibling rivalry. Envious feelings experienced by some children towards their parents in this way, or feelings experienced by the first child who envies younger siblings, will be stored away in the psyche without ever being integrated into the personality. Hence the development of two parts of us. Later on in life, when these children reach maturity and become adults, or have the opportunity to be parents themselves, they will then envy, within themselves, their own capacity to establish harmonious relationships for long enough to produce children.

I am reminded here of a man I will describe in more detail in the chapter on womb envy (see page 36). I was asked to assess him by his GP after he insisted that his pregnant young wife have a termination, on two separate occasions, on the grounds that he had made a mistake in marrying her. He had told her originally that he wanted children and they had discussed the possibility even before they married. His history was that he had envied his younger siblings so much, throughout his developmental years, that the thought of a child taking away his wife's attention sent him into a murderous rage.

Self-envy is more common than was previously thought. It comes to light only when those individuals who harbour this internal drama in their psyche are expected to behave responsibly in a two-person relationship. How many times have you heard someone say about a particular social gathering, 'He had to go and spoil it!'

As is well known in the world of psychotherapy, it is not just the other who is detested but also the very concept of a link between two people. British psychoanalyst Wilfred Bion referred to the notion of 'attacks on linking', suggesting that attacks on meaningful relationships are characteristic of envy.[1] Relationships that involve a high degree of dependency lend themselves especially easily to envious attacks.

Another way of thinking about self-envy is to visualize an internal envier who sabotages the person's interactions with significant others. This can show itself as an attack on the conceptualization of thought. A patient may say, 'I've lost my train of thought.' This can also be the case with patients suffering from self-envy – and they do suffer – who break off therapy during a positive phase rather than when they are going through a negative phase. A note I received in one particular case simply said, 'Something inside me is broken and it cannot be fixed … Therefore there is no point coming back. You have been very helpful.'

In another case, a 57-year-old male would often forget that he had a therapy session with me in another part of the hospital. He was heard to say, in a voice that could pickle fish, 'I would rather cut my throat to the bone than let that Polledri woman help me!'

Perhaps the worst and most tragic case was when a 27-year-old woman attempted suicide on Valentine's Day, a week after her fiancé of five years had asked her to marry him and have his babies. She begrudgingly said, 'How can I be expected to do that? I do not have a picture in my head of a lively mum and dad.' When I asked her once to describe what was there, she said, 'Badness in me and deadness in her … a crazy mother who disappears and a dad who is a closed book. You really cannot help me with this. I would only repeat that appalling experience if I had a baby. How ghastly!' She said she felt trapped in a black hole of hopelessness. Shortly after the first attempt, the young woman did end her life, leaving her fiancé, her family and the group of professionals consulted by them in order to help her in utter despair.

In my experience with individuals who harbour this self-envious pocket within their personality, psychotherapeutic treatment, where two individuals engage in a relationship to work through earlier unresolved experiences, has the opposite effect to what usually happens. It only stirs up, in the room, the memory of an absent thinking, listening mother who was not there to keep them in mind during their developmental years. Or, as my professor once observed, 'You are offering this person the very thing they have never had, which is deeply entrenched within their young psyche. You are someone who is there for them, but sadly they don't know how to use it to their advantage, so they have to attack it and reject the experience.'

It seems impossible for any healthy two-person relationship to develop therapeutically in this case, as the person harbouring a self-envious pocket is attached, deep within, to a self-destructive relationship that represents a lack of the life force. Their healthy, outgoing, lively part is constantly being attacked by an internal saboteur, who represents the failure they experienced, as an infant, in bonding. In that vein, the historical past is repeated, unwittingly, in the present, whether that be in therapy or in their personal relationships.

This phenomenon has been beautifully described by British psychotherapist Warren Colman as follows:

> ... *since the destructive organization is an* internal *structure, it operates not only against others, devaluing them, but also against the self, attacking and destroying any good experiences which are taken in. This maintains a sense of a lack of another within the compass of the self, which is the source of the envious person's feeling of having something missing at the core of their being.*[2]

Let me unravel this a little more. Self-envy, the turning of destructiveness against the self, is a very important situation to be aware of and understand in others, especially if you have a loved one who is prone to trying to spoil things in your life. The destructive part of that person can envy the relationship the healthy part of that person is having with you, their loved one. The idea of a happy twosome in a harmonious relationship cannot be tolerated for long and is relentlessly attacked, albeit periodically, leaving you wondering, in a very confused way, what you have done wrong. The destructive part then fizzles out for a while, you feel relieved and peace reigns … until the next time. Sadly, that is the pattern.

My only advice to you, if you are in this sort of relationship, is to remove yourself from it! Self-envy will be deeply entrenched within that person's personality and the dynamic is very resistant to treatment in therapy.

It would be comforting to think that one could turn to the literature on self-envy to discover some insight or some practical help. Unfortunately, the situation regarding the existence of an envious, destructive inner self has become increasingly confused, with an enormous muddle around definitions of the term. Basically, though, what is clear is that disruptions in early nurturing play a major part in some people's developing personality and they simply cannot bear to allow the healthy self to have any meaningful and lasting relationship with or dependency on another. This is what is underneath the impulse to sever links, in a compulsive way, with anything creative and positive in everyday life.

For example, I once treated a very talented young lady who designed beautiful period costumes for the Royal Opera House in London. Much of the time she spent hacking the finished robes to pieces and tearing up her drawings, thus delaying the production date for a particular ballet or opera.

I have known people who suffer from self-envy to fear the evil eye and turn it on themselves. When success is on the horizon, they suffer from some sort of breakdown because they cannot cope with the prospect. The success in question could be a marriage, which they will break off, saying they are not ready to commit and settle down, or the advent of a child, as in the case of the man who insisted his wife have a termination. It could also apply to the purchase of a house, when they will lie in their mortgage application, only to be turned down; or to the publication of a book, when they miss the deadline for delivering their manuscript; or professional recognition, when they fail to turn up for a final exam. Many forms of success are often followed by a period of isolation and retreat. One man I worked with would send texts saying, 'I'm sorry, I have gone into self-imposed solitary confinement' after fairly productive stages in his therapy and then disappear for months.

Some people never recover. Others restrict their achievements, as mentioned above, by sabotaging any progress with or fulfilment of their plans. The fear of success originates in the fear of the envy that success may occasion in others. Anybody who has been in the presence of such behaviour usually walks away from the situation in despair, scratching their head in bewilderment and confusion, for it never makes sense. What follows tends to be a period of envious guilt, as the person holds himself responsible for a malevolent spoiling attack on another person and then, to make matters worse, punishes himself by becoming morose. This is a very perplexing but common situation.

CHAPTER 5

ENVY AND PERVERSE BEHAVIOUR

If we are to make sense of envy and perverse behaviour, it is important to also understand that the 'other' is experienced instrumentally, becoming an object to be used rather than a subject to be known. *Hence the inherent subjectivity of the other is actively attacked in the perverse relation. But it is not just the other who is attacked. The subjectivity of self is also destroyed.*

SUSAN LONG, *THE PERVERSE ORGANISATION*
AND ITS DEADLY SINS, 2008

TO DATE, VERY little attention has been paid to envy as it is linked to perverse behaviour. This is a situation that needs to be remedied, as envy introduces a valuable element into our understanding of the genesis of psychopathology – the study of mental disorders with the aim of explaining and describing aberrant behaviour, psychopathology being the collective symptoms of a mental disorder. Envy can result in greed or refusal to take in good experiences, with unconscious violent attacks on the source of them. Since it is essentially anti-life and anti-reality, it has great explanatory value for borderline, perverse and psychotic states of mind and has proved enormously important in the analysis of destructive forces within the individual's personality.[1]

I would suggest that perversion can be a component of envy and represents the outcome of a breakdown of communication between the self and the other in relation to important figures we experience during our nurturing years. When child abuse, neglect and deprivation form part of our nurturing experience, it does not always necessarily finish us off, but it can crush our spirit. We may become victims of post-traumatic stress disorder as a result, at which point the self goes into survival mode. We all have a surviving self, which is what makes us so successful as a species – the fight or flight response, for example. However, in later life, when harmful nurturing has formed part of an individual's character structure, any loving, caring or interdependent expectations in a relationship are devalued, attacked and destroyed with pleasure.

I use the word 'perverse' to refer to a twisting or perversion of the truth. The relationship between this perversity and actual sexual perversion is not always apparent. In much of the literature, it has been recognized that a fragile ego – also called a narcissistic injury – due to childhood deprivation and abuse may trigger off envious feelings towards others who have had a 'good enough' upbringing. All of these unsatisfactory experiences are laced with shame and the urgent need this generates to keep such painful feelings out of conscious awareness. The role of perversion here puts shame in its place. It also serves as 'being in control' in a relationship. An attachment to alcohol, drugs or pornography is an unreliable one, but you can pick it up when you want it and put it down when you have finished, so you remain in control of that substance, even if not of your addiction. However, you are never in total control of another person.

In child abuse, there can be an element of envy of the child's innocence, which, of course, is ruined by abuse for ever. Yet again, the significance of shame and low self-esteem, due to early abuse and severe deprivation, creates a perverse way of relating in order to survive and be in control in a relationship. This is defensive behaviour and is far safer than risking having a healthy dependent attachment to another based on love.

Envy hides shame, which is already well concealed anyway, and acting it out in perverse behaviour keeps it under control. This destructive, narcissistic behaviour shows itself in individuals who display behaviour patterns throughout their lives that are based on a rejection and harming of the worlds of those with whom they come into contact and form intense relationships. They put all their energy into being sadistically strong by withholding their affection, thus disappointing their loved ones' attempts to enjoy any mutual, loving and sexually healthy interactions. They also regard any love in themselves as a sign of weakness.

The person who has been devalued does not need to be envied any more.

CHAPTER 6

WOMB ENVY

SO LITTLE WAS known about envy of the womb that I devoted several years of research to the subject in order to develop some understanding of this bizarre behaviour towards women.

Feminists have argued that it is the privileges of men in society that are envied, rather than the penis – as described by Freud in his theory of 'penis envy' – as such. Equally, the biological and societal privileges of women who give birth and feed and nurture their babies increase men's envy of women. For it is the difference here that arouses envy, especially if it is one upon which we depend. Womb envy denotes the envy men feel towards a woman's primary role in nurturing and sustaining life. I have often wondered how a clinician as astute as Freud, the father of psychoanalysis, could have ignored or missed the significance of such a concept as womb envy in his extensive writings over a period of fifty years.

In traditional psychoanalytic theory, women have been described as wanting the penis/phallus and the power it symbolizes. However, much less has been said about men's desire for women's 'power' of pregnancy and childbirth and its effects on the psychic well-being of men and women and society at large.[1] In coining the term, and being the first woman to challenge Freud's theory of penis envy, the psychoanalyst Karen Horney (1885–1952) proposed that men experience womb envy more powerfully than women experience penis envy because 'men need to disparage women more than women need to disparage men'.[2] Horney considered womb envy a cultural, psychosocial tendency, like the concept of penis envy, rather than an innate male psychological trait. In his 2000 book *Eve's Seed*, the historian Robert McElvaine extended Horney's argument that womb envy is a powerful, elementary factor in the psychological insecurity suffered by many men. He coined the term Non-Menstrual Syndrome, denoting a man's insecurity before the biological and reproductive powers of woman. Thus womb envy impels men to define their identities in opposition to women. Men who are envious of a woman's power to reproduce insist that a 'real man' must be 'not-a-woman', so they need to dominate women socially – by determining what women may and may not do in life – as psychological compensation for what men cannot do biologically. According to research into domestic violence undertaken by the British psychotherapist Adam Jukes, 50 per cent of abuse towards women occurs during pregnancy and continues long after the children are born.[3]

In my clinical work, I see many examples of this sort of behaviour. To go into more detail with a case I've already touched upon, I was once asked to assess a 25-year-old pregnant woman in order for her GP to justify a request for a termination on psychological grounds. She had recently married and it emerged that, for her husband, her role was to provide sexual excitement and food for him. When she became pregnant, which she said they had discussed, planned and indeed looked forward to, he insisted that she have a termination shortly before it would be illegal for her to do so under UK law. Her husband's rationale for hoping that the GP and I would agree to this was that he had made 'a terrible mistake' in marrying her and that she should return to her country of origin, as the marriage was not working out for him. Unfortunately, I did not know enough about womb envy at the time, nor about her husband's history, as she was my patient. It only later became apparent that he was destructively enacting an unresolved trauma: his encapsulated childhood anger and hatred towards his own mother for 'abandoning' him when she became severely depressed after he and his two younger siblings were born. His envy manifested itself in his intent to destroy the happiness of his young wife. It was painful and confusing for her to come to terms with his 'disappoint-ment in her' – so much so that he had convinced her that she was not 'good enough' to have his baby. Nor would he allow her to mix socially with his friends and family, completely isolating her from any interac-tion with them. His rationale for this was that they were 'disappointed by the fact that he had married a foreign girl'. Much later on, I learned by pure chance that when she became pregnant a second time, he again changed his mind, insisting that she have another termina-tion.[4]

I asked to see them as a couple, in the hope that I could shed some light on the possibility that he might have unresolved childhood expe-riences he was acting out within his marriage. He attended the appoint-ment on his own, saying that his wife would not be able to follow the conversation (in fact her English was very good). After making a de-tailed assessment of his family history, I began to suggest to him the possibility that he might be repeating his own sibling rivalry towards his unborn baby, to which he angrily replied, 'Sibling bloody warfare, you mean!' When I asked him to consider whether the unresolved con-flict within the relationship he had with his mother might also be one of the reasons he was reluctant for his wife to become a mother, his re-sponse was, 'I can't remember what you just said as I was too preoccu-pied with looking at your breasts.'

Was this a longing for the lost nurturing breast from his childhood, or an attack on my mind?

This is an example of womb envy, an envy of the creative capacity of women. Current psychiatric literature includes much more material on the crises that it is not uncommon for men to suffer when their wives or lovers are pregnant, including depressive and suicidal tenden-cies, or extreme aggressivity and hostility, which can be used as a de-fence to cover a sense of inferiority.[5] As British psychotherapist Susan Long has suggested, 'Whereas hate may wish to destroy the other, womb envy wishes to spoil and destroy the very quality that is envied.'[6]

In terms of contemporary culture, the very idea of womb envy may reflect the resentment caused by the improvement in the social position of women, who have, over the last forty years, moved into areas traditionally associated with masculinity, generally experiencing an increase in status. Conversely, when men have entered areas traditionally associated with women, such as childcare and domesticity, and have been emotionally open to nurturing, they run the risk of losing status, in their own and others' eyes, because femininity continues to be of low cultural status. This may have resulted from the fact that women no longer relate to their traditional feminine roles of passivity, vulnerability and lack, set alongside social and economic changes that mean they no longer need to be in men's care and protection as much as they used to.

A woman who thinks for herself and speaks her mind, who does not see herself as 'lacking' (a penis or anything else), effectively throws the lack back on to men, which may then threaten some of them with psychic death. Womb envy may or may not be the origin of male domination, but, according to many researchers, it is a powerful motor driving male domination.[7]

Joseph Berke explores the intense hostility that female potency and the womb generate for men (as well as other women). He argues that it may be more prevalent than penis envy, tracing the history of hatred of the womb's function in pregnancy and childbirth. His view is that 'what most women want is to be women'. He explores the parameters of such hatred in order to redress the balance of analytic thinking, concluding, 'What has been inappropriately termed *penis envy* may be more appropriately recognized and acknowledged as *womb envy*.'[8]

In the literature, male envy of female sex characteristics and reproductive capacity is a widespread and conspicuously ignored dynamic. Envy and hatred are defensively dealt with by depreciating and devaluing women. The question arises as to whether envy and devaluation of women are confined to those individuals with severe psychopathology, as in the husband I have just described, or are a more widespread dynamic in the male population. This subject is a pervasive one, expressed in the institutionalized values regarding gender and cultures universally. I believe that the envy–devaluation constellation is reflected in the selection of which traits, qualities, behaviour and roles are deemed appropriate for each sex.

Like all envy, womb envy can never be out in the open. Secretive, scheming, Machiavellian, behind the scenes, it is especially malignant because the destruction it engenders is directed at what is seen as desirable, not bad. It is this feature that is at risk of being neglected when envy is considered simply as an aspect of aggressive conflict. For womb envy to qualify as such, it has to have an undercurrent of malevolence.

Berke refers to the womb as 'the core of female potency. It is a part of the body that is perfectly placed to be idealized and envied for feeding and breeding, for loving and being made love to. Although it tends to receive a lot of the ardour and anger that may be initially directed towards the breast … the womb is far from a passive organ.'[9] It also stirs up the most uncontrollable rage in a certain category of man who feels he had no control whatsoever over his mother or the babies she made. He in turn subjects his female partner to the most violent abuse during pregnancy and continues to punish her for the loss of that most treasured of all experiences: the loving tenderness the infant is entitled to receive from its mother, of which he felt severely deprived – thus setting up a cycle of injustice, brooding, envy and destructive murderousness. According to Jukes, envy is a very potent element in men's hatred of women.

In July 2008, the press reported a case in which a man had fed his young pregnant wife a cocktail of drugs designed to cause an abortion by hiding them in her food. Eleven weeks into the pregnancy, the father of the baby (a chef by profession) had crushed an abortion pill into a sandwich he prepared for her breakfast. Within an hour, his wife was experiencing stomach cramps and bleeding, and feared that she was having a miscarriage. After he had called an ambulance and 'caringly' tried to reassure her on the way to the hospital that she would be all right, it was eventually confirmed that she had not miscarried after all. Fearing now that the baby would be 'deformed' by the pill, the next morning the husband laced a yoghurt with another abortion-inducing tablet, which he had bought on the internet. The same reaction occurred again: hospitalization with immense stomach cramps and bleeding. His wife left him after he confessed his actions to a psychologist, who insisted he told his wife the truth. He then spent days camping out on her doorstep, begging her to have a termination in case the baby was 'damaged'. He was sent to prison and, eventually, his wife gave birth to a healthy baby.

In womb envy, behind the resentment of the female partner and the need to destroy and spoil anything good that might come from a relationship, lies unconscious identification with the originally hated and needed mother or carer. Womb envy may be considered as both the source of a very basic, primitive form of hatred and a complication of the hatred that derives from the fixation of trauma. The American psychiatrist Otto Kernberg, famous for his research into borderline personality disorders, puts this very succinctly:

> *In my experience, primitive hatred takes the form of an effort to destroy the potential for a gratifying human relationship and for learning something of value in that human reaction. Underlying the need to destroy reality and communication in intimate relationships is both conscious and unconscious envy of the good object [person], particularly of an object [person] not dominated from within by similar hatred.*[10]

This explains why the husband mentioned earlier who wanted his wife to terminate her pregnancies was so full of hidden resentment and murderous rage.

To illustrate just how complicated and perplexing these experiences are for the clinician to unravel, and to emphasize the responsibility one feels towards the person on the *receiving* end of such destructive, envious and murderous behaviour, I will provide another clinical example.

After more research, I was able to decipher the underlying psychodynamics of womb envy in a case that was referred to me by a GP, as he needed a psychiatric assessment of a 32-year-old, recently divorced mother whose ex-husband wanted sole custody of the children on the grounds that she was an unfit mother. The mother had already undergone an independent assessment, arranged by her ex-husband, but the GP wanted a second opinion. Both the GP and the previous psychiatric report had, in fact, described the woman as a calm, loving and caring mother to her two daughters, one three years old and the other eleven months. She and her family, successful professional people, tried to allow for the fact that the father should have an ongoing relationship with his daughters after the breakdown of the marriage. Being good people, they did not want to deprive him or the children of that.

Having originally instigated divorce proceedings, the husband then took his case for total custody to the Royal Courts of Justice in London, claiming that his ex-wife was an abusive, violent woman. He was concerned that, if she were given custody of the children, she might harm them.

His ex-wife asked for help. Her ex-husband, she said, was also attempting to get her struck off her professional register, which would have ruined her career. Having accused her of being a child abuser, he then attempted to have her sectioned under the Mental Health Act as a mother unfit to be in sole charge of her children. The ex-wife even went as far as to suggest to social services that their staff should spend time observing her with her children in case she *was* a bad mother, having lost her sense of judgement. She had been referred to two psychiatrists for assessments at her ex-husband's insistence, for the purposes of a court report.

The GP was puzzled by the ex-husband's 'gentlemanly' behaviour when he went to see him, as this appeared contradictory. Since he was the family doctor (and had been throughout the wife's childhood), he had treated the wife for severe cuts and abdominal bruising during her second pregnancy. The doctor had no doubt that these were caused by her husband. This contrasted with the husband's claims about his wife. He would, in fact, self-harm and go to the same GP, playing the victim and saying, 'Look what my wife did to me.'

Prior to her referral to me for psychotherapy, the wife had been arrested by the police, detained in a cell for twenty-four hours and charged with actual bodily harm, on the evidence of the photographs the husband took of himself – though again he had harmed *himself* and then accused his wife of inflicting the injuries. (On closer medical examination, there is of course a distinct difference between self-inflicted bruising and injuries caused as a result of being struck by another.)

After the ex-husband had spent six months preparing for the court hearing, having subpoenaed the psychiatrists and the GP and asked for my clinical notes to appear in court, the judge made it clear in his summing-up that he saw through the ex-husband's manipulation, awarding sole custody and residency to the mother, with limited supervised access only for the father. One week after this 'unexpected' verdict, the ex-husband admitted himself to hospital, complaining of a rash and severe chest pains with panic attacks. Following a period of observation, he was eventually transferred to a psychiatric hospital, where, twenty-four hours later, he died suddenly in the psychiatric unit in mysterious circumstances at just thirty-five years of age.

During the build-up to the court case, the medical professionals involved in the assessment of the family all expressed concern for the father, but the police and social services were as determined as he was to remove the children from their mother's care. Her health visitor and the probation officer diagnosed postnatal depression, which they claimed her GP had failed to spot, although there was no evidence of such depression from the two recent psychiatric assessments prior to her referral for psychotherapy. All she was depressed about was the intractability of her hopeless situation!

The ex-husband's chilling comment shortly before the hearing was, 'Come what may, if it is the last thing I do when I leave this house, I'm taking those two children with me.'

His ex-wife's psychological well-being deteriorated markedly in the period leading up to the court case. The more she tried to be fair, pleading with her ex-husband to think about how the children were being affected, the more sadistic he became. She began to doubt her personal and professional judgement. She began to lose her confidence and vitality, but despite her overwhelming concern for her children, should he win the case, she never lost faith in the judicial system and was determined to fight back. The ex-husband had employed very expensive lawyers to build up a profile of his ex-wife as a 'hysterical psychopath', among other gender-specific expletives, hoping to have her discredited as a mother and in her professional capacity. His aim was to deprive her of everything that was precious to her: namely her children, her family, her career and her psychological stability.

As with every envious attack, the aim was to strip her of all of those attributes so that maybe then, in his eyes, she would have been less enviable.

In conclusion, chronic doubts about one's judgement can result from an envious attack, the envy being designed to destroy the very qualities the envious person might otherwise value and benefit from. The ex-wife's judgement and her maternalism were under siege and, just like Shakespeare's Othello, she was up against a threat that good judgement could not remedy.

Like the victim of racial or sexual prejudice, the envied person feels that their essential self is under attack, rather than some fault or virtue that can be changed or detached from one's central self. Instead, one's very hold on life, one's connection to the good, is the problem.[11]

I did not know anything about the ex-husband's early family history, but it struck me, on reflection, that he was spoiling and attacking the initial sense of goodness, which led in turn to destroying the family unit and attacking not only the babies that his wife was producing but also the body producing them. In other words, this case, to my mind, is an example of a much more serious psychopathology that underlines womb envy. The ex-wife often commented during her therapy that this was 'an attack on her femininity'. Her husband had been fairly genial and supportive during the first eighteen months of their marriage – she described him as a 'genuinely lovely guy' – but he changed dramatically when he learned that his wife was pregnant. He behaved like a 'sulking, broody boy'. He was more physically aggressive when she was pregnant and did not even visit her and the baby in hospital after his second daughter was born. He subsequently deprived her of all physical and sexual contact, accusing her of being the reason for 'the decline in his libido'. His wife discovered only much later that he was heavily reliant on pornography and regularly downloaded hard-core images from the internet.

Case histories like this are rare clinical examples of womb envy, an envy of the creative capacity of women. The decline in this young woman's self-confidence and her inability to continue to believe in what she had chosen to think of as a happy life were, I suggest, the result of her husband's envy and self-hatred, which he negated and reversed and put into her, then blaming her for his unhappiness.

In my clinical judgement, this man's behaviour towards his ex-wife and children is an example of rage fuelled by an envious narcissism, also typical in womb envy, which I will explain in the next chapter. The envier did not stop at trying to destroy his ex-wife; his aim was also to eradicate any hint of attachment in her, any remnant of love, need or longing – in his case, between mother and child and husband and wife. The thought of a twosome or a two-person duality sickened him.

As Berke has pointed out, 'Initially there may be a period of withdrawal from relationships and regression to an isolated state, but the conflict often leads to a near total cessation of feeling, thought and perception and can culminate in suicide.' [12]

Women have always been necessary in creating and sustaining life. Therefore, in an effort to ward off inferiority, men have attempted to produce life through unconventional means. The gift of giving birth and sustaining life has always been something that is bestowed upon women. The womb is the core of female potency. It is a part of the body that is perfectly placed to be idealized and envied ... for feeding and breeding, for loving and being made love to. The womb is not a passive organ. Considering that both penis envy and womb envy have biological and social components, if penis envy is taken to be envy of the physiological difference between men and women, then womb envy comes to be seen as envy, on the man's part, of a woman's physiological difference. [13]

In the Maternity Unit at the Royal Free Hospital in North London, there is, currently, a poster in the labour ward which reads as follows:

Childbirth isn't the only strain associated with pregnancy...Domestic violence often starts and increases during pregnancy.

CHAPTER 7

ENVY, NARCISSISM AND ZERO DEGREES OF EMPATHY

The envious person feels inferior rather than empty. He cannot stand to see others full of life and goodness, because he is preoccupied with his own limitations and defects. So his aim is to debunk and debase what others have. Security consists of equality of emptiness.

JOSEPH BERKE, *WHY I HATE YOU AND YOU HATE ME: THE INTERPLAY OF ENVY, GREED, JEALOUSY AND NARCISSISM IN EVERYDAY LIFE*, 2012

THE OBJECTS OF envy are the things we envy in others. We may envy another person's success, happiness, health, good looks, sunny disposition, character, knowledge, wealth, material possessions, power, title, job, status and even their freedom from enviousness![1]

It has long been the understanding that envious individuals are also extremely narcissistic and, like the psychopath, they tend to score highly in assessments for zero degrees of empathy.[2] Narcissism is a state of self-preoccupation. Originally applied to a consuming self-love, the concept has expanded to include any exclusive interest in and with oneself, especially as experienced in and through others. A narcissistic relationship is based on the use of primitive projective mechanisms as, for example, in envy. This is a process where the individuals place outside themselves and into someone else feelings or attributes which belong within, and come to view the mental image thus produced as objective reality. It has the desired effect of making them particularly aware of those things in others which they refuse to recognize in themselves. According to Joseph Berke, the envious person, in defending himself against envious tension, can easily lock himself into a narrow, self-centred existence, which is narcissism par excellence.[3] Many enviers also tend to focus on their own perceived image of the envied person, no matter how irritating or distorted, rather than take the chance of discovering someone or something in its own right.

I agree with Berke that envy and narcissism are variations of the same problem: excessive mental pain, an overwhelming sense of inferiority and feelings of inadequacy. He puts it beautifully when he states, 'To begin with the envious and the narcissistic person attack this problem differently, the envier by deflating others, the narcissist by inflating himself, but their thinking, feelings, and actions run along divergent tracks.'[4]

Narcissism can be typically defined as a perverted and pathological self-absorption and pride that interfere with or preclude relations with others, not a normal or healthy self-esteem that is the prelude to mutual respect and reciprocal exchange. This is the basis for any healthy interactive duality in a relationship. The narcissist has little or no self-esteem. Like the envier, the narcissist looks upon others with an eye that puffs them up and squashes them flat as soon as he perceives qualities or features that he considers better than his own. It is a fact that to envy somebody, the narcissist has to admire *something* in that person to begin with. Then narcissistic interest turns into envious hatred.

Narcissism begets envy. The Brothers Grimm, in their story of Snow White, vividly narrated the relationship between narcissistic failure and envy. In this instance, the awareness for the queen of another's beauty provokes a storm of narcissistic malice. The queen is no longer concerned with inflating her own ego, but aims to wreak havoc on a figure, Snow White, who has dared disturb, albeit unwittingly, her lofty reveries. She sends for a huntsman and tells him to take the child out into the forest and kill her, bringing back her lungs and liver as proof that the job's been done. She launches her attack on the actual person, on any reflection of that person and on her perception of the reflection. In the Grimm story, the queen spares the magic mirror, representing reality. In other versions of the story she smashes the mirror as well, presumably to kill off the possibility that she is no longer 'the fairest of them all'.

Greed is another characteristic that has been compared with envy, but, to continue the fairy-tale theme, the greedy person wants the golden eggs that the goose lays whereas the envious person wants to kill the golden goose so that nobody can have the eggs!

Rage, fuelled by envious narcissism, does not stop at destroying the object of envy but aims to eradicate any sort of attachment in the other.

The dysfunctional behaviours of a narcissistic personality always include:

- a grandiose sense of his importance
- phantasies of unlimited power
- thoughts of being unique and 'special'
- belief that everything is owed to him
- exploitation of others in relationships
- lack of empathy

I am reminded here of the teachings of Otto Kernberg, who points out that envy is a fundamental underlying trait in narcissistic individuals because they feel intense envy of those who seem to possess things they don't have or who are simply relaxed and find pleasure in living. In particular, he says, they don't suffer true feelings of sadness, loss or mourning, and it is this inability to experience depressive reactions that is a basic element of their personality.[5] Their driving force is envy and their objective is taking over. To envy is to covet and to feel spiteful irritation at the sight of the happiness and the advantages of other people. At the outset, we are dealing with an abusive mentality based on a perception of what the other possesses and they perceive themselves to lack. These are always the underlying psychodynamics in envious individuals.

They are more anxious to destroy the material or spiritual benefits others have than to acquire them for themselves.

ZERO DEGREES OF EMPATHY

The British neuroscientist Simon Baron-Cohen talks about three types of zero degrees of empathy: borderline, psychopath and narcissist. He does not include envy in his theory, but I believe that a fair percentage of those who score highly on the Baron-Cohen Empathy Questionnaire (EQ) scale as having zero degrees of empathy are also extremely envious individuals.

Empathy can be defined as our ability to identify with what someone else is thinking or feeling, and to respond to their thoughts and feelings with an appropriate emotion. Baron-Cohen asks, 'What does it mean to have no empathy, and does this translate into what some people call evil?' He takes old categories from psychiatry and reconceptualizes them as examples of zero degrees of empathy. For example, citing Hervey Cleckley, the expert in psychopathy, in his definition of a psychopath, Baron-Cohen argues that psychopaths – those with zero degrees of empathy – show:

- superficial charm and plausibility
- hidden anxiety and depression
- undependability and dishonesty
- egocentricity
- an inability to form lasting intimate relationships
- a failure to learn from punishment
- a poverty of emotions
- a lack of insight into the impact of their behaviour on others
- a failure to plan ahead
- passive aggression[6]

Clearly some psychopaths hurt others through physical aggression, but the breakthrough in Cleckley's formulation was to extend this concept to those who are aggressive in more subtle and sometimes under-hand ways, like passive aggression.

This is where I think the concept of envy in relation to narcissism and lack of empathy is relevant. We can assume that it makes sense to say that empathy is always lacking in the mind of the envier, but I would argue that you need a heightened sense of deviousness and intuition to consciously know how your behaviour will harm and hurt another. Especially as the envier does not want what you have for *himself*, it's just that he does not want *you* to have it.

Baron-Cohen believes that having zero degrees of empathy is ultimately a lonely kind of existence. It means that you have no brakes on your behaviour, which leaves you free to pursue any object you desire, or to express any thought in your mind, without considering the impact of your actions or words on anyone else. In extreme cases, it might even lead you to commit murder.

This is clearly another variant of envy, for among the individuals I have interviewed and assessed who have killed a loved one, none of them had any empathy whatsoever for the person, or family of that person, whose lives they had taken, except, sometimes, in a superficial way. It was interesting to note that not one of the individuals I came across had had a 'good enough' upbringing, to use the phrase coined by the British pioneer of attachment theory, Donald Winnicott.

According to the *Diagnostic and Statistical Manual of Mental Disorders*, enviousness of others is a predominant trait in narcissistic people. I would agree with Cleckley that the following characteristics are extremely relevant when considering not only psychopathic personalities but also envious, narcissistic individuals:

- unreliability
- untruthfulness and insincerity
- lack of remorse or shame
- *envy of others*
- poor judgement and failure to learn from experience
- incapacity for love

- suicide rarely carried out
- sex life impersonal and poorly integrated
- failure to follow any life plan
- lying[6]
- always the victim

After working in the field of forensic psychiatry and psychiatry with many envious, narcissistic individuals, I can assure you that envy is emotional abuse.

CHAPTER 8

ENVY IN ACADEMIA

MY FIRST EXPERIENCE of envy in academia was when a senior academic had to mark an excellent piece of work I had handed him from a female degree student who was predicted to receive a distinction. As he read it in his office, his back to me, he muttered to himself, 'I'll kill it ... I'll kill it stone dead! (He was her second supervisor.)

The information contained in this chapter did not appear in my book *Envy is Not Innate: A New Model of Thinking*. That book was based on my doctoral thesis and I had been told, when writing my thesis, that it would be unwise to antagonize the professors and examiners at the university where I completed my first chunk of research. I include it here not only because I consider it to be of great importance, but also because this remains a little-discussed issue, one nobody dares to write about it for fear of aliening those colleagues in universities and academic institutes of excellence with the power to decide whose career will flourish. The rare exception is the work of Professor Glenn Hudak in America (see Further Reading), but otherwise it is virtually impossible to find any papers related to this topic.

I also experienced this hideous envy when I was writing up my first research project, for which I had devised a maternal questionnaire to test out and diagnose a condition known as Munchausen Syndrome by Proxy. I had developed a way of working with the mothers therapeutically, as these women were ill and should not have gone to prison. I had written quite a considerable amount on the subject previously and had actually decided that it was, in fact, a perversion of the maternal instinct.

I will quote from just a few incidents that, looking back, were envious attacks on my progress.

The first was when I met one of my supervisors, Professor T. He listened carefully to my proposal and then said very sarcastically, 'Well, I can see *your* name in lights!' He then proceeded to block any progress over the next three years by his *inaction*. Examples included losing copies of my draft thesis that I had left on his desk, forgetting to turn up for tutorials and suggesting I had got the date wrong when I finally tracked him down. When I asked him, in a very frustrated manner, just how much longer it would be before I could submit the thesis for examination, he replied with an innocent smile on his face, 'How long is a piece of string?' The last straw came when he said to my second supervisor, 'How is Miss Bright Eyes doing?' She, being a fairly timid and shy person, was worried for me when I did, at her suggestion, ask for a change of supervisor. Professor T. refused to acknowledge any work I'd already done and I had to start the process all over again, with a change of supervisor, which took another three years for me to complete. Some supervision!

It has to be said that I have also experienced wonderful moments of joy, friendship and job satisfaction as an academic. But there have been times when I have felt the debilitating pain of alienation, being ignored and marginalized because others envied either my work or my enthusiasm, or both. I have also experienced my pain anew as I observed other academics on the receiving end of ruthless envy. And yet there are those who, like my last dissertation editor, willingly and generously continue to spend time helping those who are struggling to complete their research. They encourage the new to persist, they shine as beacons of hope in moments of despair and they join together with others in a common struggle to humanize the academic workplace.

But within the hierarchical structure of academia the relationship between the envier and the envied occurs not only from the bottom up but from the top down. Senior members often envy the energy, optimism, enthusiasm and insights of the newer students, or, as they are often called, 'new blood'. For those who are the object of a senior member's envy, it feels like being turned from a person into a thing, where the envier still holds all the power. I became objectified as 'Miss Bright Eyes' to Professor T.

Short of leaving all that you have worked so hard for by giving up and binning your research, as I was sometimes tempted to do out of frustration, or committing some form of academic suicide, little can be done about this sort of envy in many cases. In personal terms, as Hudak points out, 'it is as if one has become a garbage can into which tainted stuff of the envier can be dumped'.[1] Human relationships, any bond of sympathy or understanding, can be blocked ... as was the case with me and Professor T.

The envied person becomes increasingly desperate, for nothing succeeds in warding off envy. If you try to share your work or ideas, you are attacked for showing off or for being patronizing. If you try to defend yourself by explaining, you are not listened to. Envied students who try to discuss their situation are treated by others as spoiled, or whinging and complaining. So an almost total breakdown of communication occurs between envying and envied students in an environment where envy has taken hold: people hear what they want to hear and see what they want to see, remember what they want to remember and believe what they want to believe. It is a waste of time complaining.

This is, of course, an abuse of power, not supervision and encouragement of a student on their way to academic progress. We should be aware of the corrosive nature of envy in academia: how it thwarts the good and hence suffocates the impulse to cooperate. Furthermore, we need to realize that envy is widespread in our society and while we can run we cannot hide. We have to learn to play the game.

CHAPTER 9

ENVY IN THE WORKPLACE

For not many men, the proverb saith,
Can love a friend whose fortune prospereth
Unenvying; and about the envious brain
Cold poison clings and doubles all the pain
Life brings him. His own woundings he must nurse,
And feel another's gladness like a curse.

AESCHYLUS, *AGAMEMNON*

I THINK IT is a good idea to add a small section on envy as it is encountered in the workplace. Here we see management stifling the work and curbing the enthusiasm of subordinates. They stifle development to preserve their status and salary. Internal politics can be the cancer of organizations. If we think about the way workplaces and organizations are set up, it raises an interesting question: is competition the best way to get your employees to produce? It's possible, in some circumstances, that competition is good. However, if some people are preoccupied with bringing others down, that's not healthy for any organization. It is also true that envious people undervalue their own efforts while being resentfully impressed by those of others.

Envy in the workplace damages relationships, disrupts teams and undermines performance. Most of all it harms the one who feels it. When we are obsessed with someone else's success, our self-respect suffers and we may neglect or even sabotage our own performance and possibly our

50

career. Comparing ourselves with successful workmates can be motivating, but it can also trigger envy.

Such feelings may cause real damage, both to our own career and to our organization's success. Denying or concealing envy makes the problem worse. Regardless of the economic climate, people at all levels of an organization are vulnerable to envy. In the workplace, envy is difficult to manage, because it is hard to admit that we harbour such a socially unacceptable emotion. Some people become so fixated on a rival that they lose their focus on their own performance.

Envy can become a real issue for both employers and employees, dividing workforces and distracting people from the jobs they want and are paid to do. When a co-worker has something we want – for example, a better job title, salary or perks – instead of feeling pleased for them, or understanding why they are in a stronger position, we feel inferior and resent their success. This is when envy is stirred up, when we feel we are not being treated in the same way as our colleagues. This is where competition and envy clash. Competition involves wanting to outdo the other person, whereas envy is resenting what the other person has, wanting to take it away and even wishing to see the other person ruined. If our response to another's success or promotion is to channel our envy towards the other, there can be no positive consequences.

Envy in the workplace isn't pleasant. News of a colleague's good fortune can send us spiralling into a black hole of depression and weak self-righteousness. It poisons our confidence and undermines our sense of worth. But facing this 'green-eyed monster' can tell us important things about ourselves – mainly, that we need to change. Seen this way, envy can be a powerful motivator to seek professional counselling. This will point us in the right direction, to the belief that goodness is within our reach if we admit how destructive this feeling of envy is. Think of it as fuel to drive us to a better frame of mind. The task at hand here is to use that 'envy' to improve your situation instead of allowing it to intensify your hatred.

Favouritism at work certainly stirs up envy. Significant envy in our own childhood makes us particularly susceptible to it. The 'office family', with its particular hierarchy of senior adults in charge, sibling rivalry, divided resources of time, affection and money, carries echoes of our own families of origin.

Finally, envy is almost universally provoked by outstanding achievement. In an article in *Psychology Today* by Judith Sills, 'When Green is Mean' (September 2008), a journalist describes how she worked on a newspaper for years with a great group of people. But when her book became a surprise best-seller, they weren't so great any more. At least not to her. They were sniping, cold and critical of her other work. It came as a surprise to her and it hurt.

Envy in the workplace is difficult to manage. We spend some forty hours a week at work, only to go home and torment ourselves even further by conducting a post-mortem on our day. Part of this drama is to conceal or deny these feelings, and that makes things worse. Repressed envy inevitably resurfaces in a stronger form.

We are not used to talking about envy in the workplace, yet it is there, woven into the fabric of organizations. It affects the mood and morale of employees and, ultimately, it is one of the causes of employee disengagement and loss of productivity.

PART III: FORENSIC PSYCHIATRY AND THE OSCAR PISTORIUS CASE

CHAPTER 10

WHAT IS FORENSIC PSYCHIATRY AND PSYCHOTHERAPY?

THE UK WAS instrumental in pioneering a psychoanalytic understanding of criminology. At the start of the 1990s, this interest in forensic psychotherapy was given fresh impetus when forensic psychiatry was recognized as a sub-speciality of the Royal College of Psychiatrists.

The development of forensic services in the UK was linked to the study of the triggers determining the behaviour of those convicted of murder or harming a loved one that resulted in their being admitted to 'special hospitals', such as Broadmoor, Rampton and Ashworth, with therapeutic communities where they could be treated, if suitable, with psychotherapy during their sentence, to stop them reoffending or repeating their dangerous behaviour when released back into a medium-secure unit in their place of origin.

In 1992, I was the first of a small number of trainees to graduate from the initial forensic psychotherapy diploma course at the Portman and Tavistock Clinic NHS Trust, in conjunction with the British Medical Foundation. This course has developed over the past twenty years and the discipline of forensic psychotherapy has grown enormously since then. The programme developed further to include many prisoners suffering from mental disorders and abnormalities and is responsible for their discharge and aftercare, again with the aim of preventing further reoffending behaviour.

For the forensic psychotherapist, the criminal act is seen as a consequence of a state of mind in which unconscious processes and unconscious phantasy, as well as conscious thought, combine or play a key role. The recurrent question is: what is the meaning of the act?

> *Forensic psychotherapists are concerned with the psychodynamic understanding of the particular offender patient and, in this context, the actual details of the crime become important as a means to understand better the psychological profile and disturbance of the offender in relation to his or her offending behaviour. Forensic patients are unique because they demonstrate what is going on in their minds by the behaviour they act out. It seems that, in my experience, they are not able to express this verbally when they commit the crime. It is the details of the behaviour that are examined in order for the judge to decide whether the offender goes to prison or a special hospital.*[1]

The model used in forensic psychotherapy, as described by Arthur Hyatt Williams and Christopher Cordess, places particular emphasis upon the developmental importance of the experience an individual had in their first and early years, so that early failure by the carer *and* experiences of trauma or abuse are predicted to have significant psychological effects in later life.[2] Unresolved anger and resentment, for example, may explode in a way that is quite out of proportion to the provocation. They smoulder away inside, like an unexploded bomb, and are detonated by an external trigger.

In forensic psychotherapy it is not unusual to meet people who routinely carry a lethal weapon, rationalizing it as being 'for the purposes of self-defence'. Underlying such rationalization there may be the thought or phantasy: 'If I am threatened I can and I will kill.' Or a previous, emotionally unbearable, traumatic experience may erupt into offensive action if it has been 'split off' and, psychologically speaking, remained 'undigested' or 'unmetabolized'. When there are later psychological stresses – either external, such as the threat of the loss of a loved one, or intra-psychic, such as depression or a paranoid illness –

then the previously stable, internal situation may explode, so that the individual feels 'taken over' by the external situation.

This is the background against which I intend to consider the Oscar Pistorius case.

CHAPTER 11

OSCAR PISTORIUS: AN EXAMPLE OF ENVY IN ACTION

A heart at peace gives life to the body, but envy rots the bones.

PROVERBS 14:30

OSCAR PISTORIUS

THIS FAMOUS SOUTH African athlete, also known as the Blade Runner, is a six-times Paralympic gold medallist and the first double amputee in history to compete in the Olympic Games alongside able-bodied athletes. He was born in Johannesburg in 1986 with fibular hemimelia, meaning that he had no fibula – the long, thin bone that extends from the ankle to the knee and supports the full weight of the body – in either leg. This is the most common form of lower-limb deficiency at birth. It is commonly the case that the foot is not sufficiently formed and is best amputated through the ankle, and an artificial limb is usually fitted eventually. The decision was taken by Pistorius's parents to have his legs amputated from the knee downwards when he was eleven months old. The surgeon was convinced that if the double amputation was performed before the baby learned to walk, he would never know what it was like to walk on his own feet and so would not suffer the trauma of having lost them. Having overcome his disability, through sheer determination and ambition to be just the same as everybody else, Pistorius went on to become known as 'the fastest man on no legs'.

On Valentine's Day 2013, he shot and killed 29-year-old Reeva Steenkamp, a beautiful, vivacious model and his girlfriend of just twelve weeks. He was acquitted of premeditated murder but convicted on the lesser charge of culpable homicide, the South African term for manslaughter. He was also found guilty of a separate firearms charge and was sentenced to five years in prison. This verdict is currently being challenged by the Supreme Court of Appeal by the prosecution in order for it to be upgraded to murder.

BACKGROUND HISTORY

This case provides a good example of how the complicated dynamics of envy – which, as we have seen, is not innate – can emerge and develop, due to external circumstances, throughout a child's upbringing.

In a spirit of compassionate understanding, Oscar Pistorius's life can be seen as unfolding against a stark backdrop of loss and deprivation. It is important to describe the very difficult circumstances of his early life and to envisage a perfect little boy born with a disability. We cannot imagine what shame and embarrassment his mother may have felt giving birth to a disabled child; nor the effect on his father, who was to desert him and his two siblings when Pistorius was six years old.

The central factor in any exploration of Oscar Pistorius's personality must begin with the trauma he underwent at a pre-verbal stage of his development when both his legs were amputated from below the knee. The experience of this primary loss would have been associated with any other secondary loss he experienced throughout his life. The only information we have about the traumatic impact the amputation had is his father's recollection of visiting his baby son on the night after the operation. He found him in his cot, very distressed and screaming in pain. His father asked the nurses on duty if he had been given any medication for the pain. They told him that they did not know what dosage to give a baby under one, so they had decided not to medicate at all.

The furious father phoned the surgeon, who arrived from his home in pyjamas and gave the baby some pain relief.

Having consulted with a number of experts, Pistorius's parents managed the amputation as well as could be expected and worked hard to ensure that their son's post-operative experience was as painless as possible. He was fitted with prosthetic legs when he was fourteen months old so that he could learn to walk. What is clear is that from then on he was not allowed to show any vulnerability, and this would, no doubt, have facilitated the development of a deep-rooted and suppressed trauma which would have affected his growing sense of self. The stage was set for him to prove he was as able-bodied as anyone else.

His mother, Sheila, played a pivotal role in working relentlessly to ensure that he would never see himself as being different. That she was key in the development of his determination to be able to adjust physically and functionally is something that Pistorius speaks about on a regular basis, which suggests an idealization of his mother and his deep gratitude to her for all that he became. He mirrored the same determination in his sporting success on the world stage that his mother displayed in response to his amputation. He had his mother's dates of birth and death tattooed on his forearm.

In his book *The Blade Runner*, Pistorius talks about how the news that his parents were getting divorced was 'a serious and sudden blow'. They had to sell their house and the children moved with their mother to a smaller one nearer town. Life as he knew it was never the same again for him and his siblings. His father moved 700 miles away to Port Elizabeth – as chance would have it, the city where Reeva Steenkamp grew up. His father did not meet all of his financial responsibilities afterwards and his mother had to go to work. They went from being a well-off white family, in a country where to be born white had always been a guarantee of material security, to a family in which every penny counted.

Sheila Pistorius had no intention of enrolling her son in any kind of special school for children with disabilities. He went to a regular primary school. Aged fourteen, he chose to go to Pretoria Boys' High School, which had a military element to its culture. In the interview he and his mother had with the headmaster for a place at this boarding school, which was paid for by his uncle, the headmaster verbalized his concerns as to whether or not the young Oscar would be able to cope. His mother looked baffled and replied, 'I don't think I follow. What are you saying?' When the headmaster mumbled something about the boy's condition, his ... er ... prosthetic legs, she replied, 'Ah, I see, but please don't worry. There is no problem at all. He is absolutely normal.'[1]

Although he had an able-bodied older brother and younger sister to protect him during his younger years, later, at boarding school, he was subjected to bullying. Aged thirteen, some boys in his dormitory lit a fire by spraying lighting fluid on to a metal cabinet behind his bed. They then hid his prosthetic legs and left him to escape on his stumps. Everyone was told to evacuate the building. Panic-stricken, he frantically searched everywhere for his prosthetics, as they were not where he left them. Terrified and in tears, he became hysterical, afraid that he would be left to die. The boys carried on laughing at the fright they had given him, long after the flames were extinguished. Yet, although he never reported the incident to his housemaster, years after he left school, when he was famous, he never stopped mentioning the incident in one interview after another. He shrugged it all off, presenting himself as a good sport, capable of taking a joke.

Here we see the beginning of the development of a sense of injustice, so common in envious individuals, which I will go on to describe in more detail later. What is crucial to consider in terms of his psychological make-up at this point, though, is that his mother failed to see that by hiding the truth from himself and others, he might gain in his self-image in the short term but lose out ultimately by failing to face up to the reality of his disabled body, thus hampering his capacity to develop as an emotionally healthy human being.

Was this the beginning of his ability to deny totally the truth in any situation: namely, details of what happened on the night he shot Reeva Steenkamp?

Another element to this story is the uncomfortable truth that Pistorius failed to register that his mother often drank herself to sleep. She was an intermittent and solitary alcoholic who found relief from the pain of the reality she feared to confront in a bottle.[2]

His next major trauma was the death of his mother after a short but misdiagnosed illness when he was fifteen years old. He describes feeling like a rudderless boat in the aftermath. It is clear that there was no support system to help the young Pistorius to cope after his mother's death. Adults, coaches and teachers who tried to help him at different stages could never have replaced his mother's nurturing and her fierce determination that he was to be treated just the same as everyone else.

After the loss of his mother, Pistorius chose to fend for himself and so, at the age of seventeen, having graduated from Pretoria Boys' High School, he set up home alone. This is another example of his self-sufficiency and his over-developed qualities of determination and competitiveness. However, the flipside to this sort of behaviour would have been an intolerance of frustration and being guarded in his emotions. He would not have been able to trust easily in relationships. Closeness and intimacy would have been a fearful prospect so to avoid them would have been paramount; the alternative was to enter into multiple relationships in order to protect himself from becoming overly attached and to act out obsessively. It was at this stage of his development that he became obsessed with firearms.

Throughout interviews once he became famous as a seventeen-year-old sprinter he made reference to the fact that he was not disabled. He proceeded to start a legal case against the International Association of Athletics Federations to be allowed to enter competitions as an able-bodied runner. Here we see an all-consuming mission to be regarded as normal. He appears to have lost touch with the realities surrounding his disability. His determination was to fulfil his mother's legacy in showing the world that he was able and equal in all aspects of life. Here again we see an extreme element of denial. But his self-esteem would have been dependent on reassurance from the external world, which, by their awards and applause, fulfilled the same role as his mother. He would have worked even harder for external validation to increase his self-esteem. It is clear from his behaviour in late adolescence that his self-esteem was dependent on his ability to achieve in order to neutralize his disability.

He always pushed himself way beyond normal expectations to be the best, the fastest, the most admired in his field. But what was going on inside must have been very different. Being disabled made him famous, but it must have been very painful to acknowledge that he spent most of his life trying so hard to be normal. One wonders whether there was any space at all for him to show any vulnerability or weakness. There were many waiting in line for a piece of his lucrative success. His father only started to take an interest in him again after he became famous.

Pistorius's craving to be accepted must also have been extended to his relationships with women. In all of his relationships he demanded the unconditional nurturing love his mother had lavished on him. He would, on one level, idealize these perfect, loving, blonde women, but when they fell short of perfection, he would reject and betray them. On the outside he was being crowned with glory for his sporting achievements, but when he was alone, having to remove his prosthetic legs, he would have to confront his deformity and imperfections.

Prior to the death of Reeva Steenkamp, Pistorius had been through some of the most challenging times of his life: the mental and physical preparations for the 2012 London Olympics. It is clear, though, from the account given by Trisha Taylor, the mother of his girlfriend before Reeva Steenkamp, that the emotional and obsessive calls he made to the family during the build-up to the event were a sign of his psychological deterioration. Pistorius had made a mess of his relationship with Samantha Taylor and, in an attempt to move on, she became involved with someone else. All this unfolded while Pistorius was in London, competing in the Olympics, and his inability to control the situation from afar sent him over the edge. Trying and failing to win back Samantha Taylor may well have influenced the possessive way he behaved in his new relationship some months later with Reeva Steenkamp. This might, perhaps, shed some light on what led up to and contributed to the tragedy for which he was to become notorious.

(It is worth reading Patricia Taylor's book, *Oscar: An Accident Waiting to Happen*, which gives a very revealing account of how much trouble Pistorius caused her family during the relationship he had with her daughter.[3])

Sadly, in the London Olympics Pistorius had not achieved what he set out to do: to prove to the world that he could compete with and beat the best athletes. Additionally, he not only failed to win his 200-metre race in the Paralympics, but he lost his cool when he was beaten. When he came second to Alan Oliveira, the Brazilian blade runner, Pistorius publicly accused Oliveira of cheating, claiming that his blades were longer, thus improving his stride. This was later found to be untrue.

As Carlin describes, for Pistorius a pattern repeated itself in relationships time and again, from petulant possessiveness to frantic dependency, to hysterical fear of loss. No one could quite measure up. He could not help himself when jealousy consumed him and he saw rivals everywhere. But he was a man of extremes, which added a uniquely corrosive edge to his insecurities about love and sex. The blade runner and the private Oscar Pistorius were in perpetual conflict.

Running became his refuge from any conflict in his personal life. Pistorius subjected himself to a strict training regime in an attempt to keep his anxiety in check. The younger Oscar was coerced into living a lie that declared he was able-bodied. He had no experience of empathy, no doubt because his family thought of his disability as 'a pity', which, as stiff puritanical Boers, they shunned.

Patricia Taylor speaks poignantly when she describes how she welcomed Pistorius into her family with open arms, but she goes on to show how he was unable to fit in and be part of the family:

> *On a certain level, even though Oscar seemed to thrive being part of our family, I am sure that all of that closeness we expressed towards each other might have been too much for him to handle; pushing certain buttons that created deep feelings of inadequacy and resentment. While outwardly he bonded with us, and he experienced real happiness being part of the family, he also confessed a number of times that he felt envious of the family and the closeness we enjoyed. And he admitted to us that there was something*

inside him that made him do stupid, self-destructive things, especially when everything was going well.

She describes many incidents which illustrate his envy in action, when his perplexing behaviour ruined many otherwise happy family gatherings. She also found it strange that although he stayed with them many times, he would never bring a thing, not a slab of chocolate or a bottle of wine, as most people would when visiting. He didn't seem to be able to think beyond his own needs.

I often wondered what effect all of these perfect beautiful women he always dated had on Oscar, given his disability. Maybe deep down, all of them in some way made Oscar feel his own disability more acutely, which might, in the end, have driven him over the edge. Maybe all his desperate attempts to control them and treat them like inanimate objects were all because somewhere their perfection reminded him too much of the imperfections within himself. [4]

When I read about this tragedy, I was reminded of a young woman I once treated for depression after she had been in a ten-year marriage with a disabled man who often used a wheelchair due to the disability he was born with. He chose as a partner a beautiful, sweet-natured young woman, from a loving family, who devoted herself to him to prove she loved him, and that his disability did not matter to her. When she came to therapy, she did so in order to save her own sanity. He would constantly pick on her, create scenes in front of her friends, criticize her for the way she spoke and spoil social occasions by accusing her of flirting with able-bodied men. He manipulated her feelings to destroy her life. What he envied most was her peace of mind and the absence of envy. Basically, he took a kind, loving girl from a strong, secure family and returned a broken woman to them ten years later. It would appear that the family of Samantha Taylor experienced the same dilemma.

Returning to Pistorius, from his developmental history one can see how easily he would fit into the role of an adult behaving in a very envious way towards someone he originally admired. For to envy someone you have to admire them first. He would then have been unable to deal with the resulting frustration for fear of vulnerability. His behaviour, when confronted emotionally in a relationship, would have been violent and destructive and self-damaging in the face of challenges and conflict. He would have been very sensitive to rejection and would have had an urge to control whoever he was in a relationship with, in order to resta-bilize his self-esteem.

REEVA STEENKAMP

Reeva Steenkamp's developmental history was totally the opposite to that of Oscar Pistorius. Young, beautiful and full of life, she was someone who cared deeply for others and who was loved by her family and friends. She was a successful model and her television career was about to take off, as she was due to make her debut as a fledgling television presenter in South Africa. She also had a law degree. It is exactly this type of indi-vidual who can seem very enviable to those with a less fortunate back-ground and family history, such as Pistorius.

Words used to describe Reeva by her close friends and family in-cluded 'intelligent', 'vivacious', 'classy', 'generous of spirit', 'kind', 'funny', 'witty', 'humble', 'selfless', 'caring', 'gentle', 'loyal', 'strong-willed', 'a champion of women's rights', 'consistent', 'amazing', 'socially engaging' and 'a child of God'.

As we have seen, to envy somebody you have to admire them first, and this was what happened when Oscar Pistorius asked a friend to in-troduce him to Reeva Steenkamp, having first seen a picture of her on the cover of a magazine.

Here the object is not jealousy, but a tormenting sense of doubt, dis-trust or suspicion regarding the faithfulness of a beloved person – envy as a feeling of bitterness and vexation provoked by someone else's success and well-being. It is a spontaneous desire to destroy what one person has on the part of another person who feels they have been deprived. And, tragically, complete integrity can be destroyed only by destroying the body.

It may well be that the court failed Reeva Steenkamp and her family by denying them justice in the sentencing of Oscar Pistorius. But by not understanding the pathology of envy, and the severe psychological disturbance that it is, we fail as an intellectual community. The dynamic here is that the envious person always destroys what is good in someone else; they do not seem to concern themselves with unhappy, nasty or aggressive individuals.

Devaluation of an envied person is a typical manoeuvre, for as long as the envied is being devalued, he or she need not be envied. Otto Kernberg taught us this in his work with borderline and narcissistic patients, when he said that intense envy and hatred of women are easy to spot because they spoil the capacity to form and maintain loving relationships. He found that envy and hatred are defensively dealt with by depreciating and devaluing women.[5] In the evidence gathered by the prosecution, Reeva Steenkamp told her close friends that Pistorius always seemed to be angry with her, even from the very early stages of their brief, twelve-week relationship. Reeva's mother remembered a phone call she had from Reeva one night while she was in a car with Pistorius. She was very frightened because he was driving at a dangerously high speed. She asked her mother to tell him to slow down. That was the only conversation June Steenkamp ever had with Pistorius. Reeva also told her mother and friends that they argued a lot.

A SENSE OF INJUSTICE

The envious person's sense of injustice is based on a feeling of resentment. This sense of injustice is necessary for hostile feelings to emerge as it is part of the envious response. To an envious person, the envied other 'has it all' – good looks and brains. But the crowning advantage is that they are also *good* people. As Reeva Steenkamp was described as being. Their goodness does not lessen the intensity of the hostile envy; rather, it only fuels it! Understanding hostile envy seems particularly important, because such feelings have the obvious potential to destroy social interaction. An envious person *always* claims there is injustice in his life, real or imagined, to warrant such spiteful, envious behaviour.

In Pistorius's case, as mentioned earlier, he complained of injustice when he came second in a race at the London Olympics in 2012, falsely accusing the winner of cheating. During the trial he complained of injustice because the crime scene on the night was tampered and interfered with by the police. Yet he interfered with every aspect of the crime scene itself. He interfered with the toilet door by bashing it in with a cricket bat after he fired the shots. He interfered with Reeva's mobile phone, the contents of the toilet bowl and, not least, Reeva's body by carrying her downstairs and removing her from the crime scene.

As a display of his narcissism, during the trial Pistorius said, 'I felt trapped.' (Reeva was trapped in the toilet.)

Pistorius said, 'I was frightened.' (Reeva was terrified and screaming, based on evidence from several ear-witnesses.)

Pistorius said, 'I felt vulnerable.' (Yet he was standing with a loaded weapon, the bullets being the highly destructive black talon rounds, and he was in his own house, in a secure complex with an alarm system.)

Pistorius said, 'I approached the bathroom to protect myself and Reeva.' (He did not need to protect himself or Reeva, as the door was locked. Yet he shot Reeva and failed to protect himself when he smashed the door down.) [6]

Another display of his narcissism in relation to envy is how Pistorius never used the word 'we' or 'us' during his trial. He says 'I'. This connection is listed in the *Diagnostic and Statistical Manual of Mental Disorders*. Here is another example of how envious people negate and reverse a situation to prove injustice, instead of taking responsibility for their own destructive behaviour. The injustice here was that Reeva may have been perceived by Pistorius as having an unfair advantage over him if she threatened to call the police or a friend for help when she fled to the bathroom, taking her mobile phone with her and locking the door.

When he shot Reeva he did not phone for an ambulance or security, he called his friends. Pistorius claimed that when he phoned the emergency services, at 3.20 a.m., he was told, 'Take Reeva to the hospital.' But you don't have to be a trained medic to appreciate that if a genuine attempt was to be made to save Reeva's life, the first priority ought to have been to stem the massive blood loss she was suffering. A layperson knows that anyone bleeding to that extent should not be moved. In fact, during the trial, it emerged that when a neighbour arrived, an ambulance had not yet been called. It was actually the neighbour who tried to stem the blood flow and called for an ambulance, not Pistorius. Nor was there any record of him phoning the emergency services.

Let's go back to the cross-examination in which he says, 'I did not intend to kill Reeva, my lady, or anybody else.'

If Pistorius did not intentionally shoot Reeva, or anyone else for that matter, then what did he intend? He simply discharged his weapon four times because he was nervous? Fired blindly at a noise he heard behind the door? Screamed at the intruder, or burglar, to 'get the fuck out of my house' and then … fired four warning shots? Reeva probably had time to scream as Pistorius fired the first shot into the locked toilet. It should be remembered that the pathologist who performed the post-mortem on her body told the court that it would have been 'unnatural' for her not to scream in agony after Pistorius fired the first shot, which shattered her hip.

The judge ruled that the state had failed to prove beyond a reasonable doubt that Pistorius knew it was Reeva when he fired four shots through the door into the toilet, where she had locked herself in with her mobile phone. The athlete's home was in an exclusive, high-security gated community in Pretoria. It had CCTV, electrified twelve-foot perimeter walls and underground sensors that ringed the complex. Uniformed guards were on constant patrol on foot with dogs, and also on bicycles, twenty-four hours a day. Throughout the trial, he insisted that he mistook his girlfriend for an intruder.

During the trial, it transpired that Reeva may have received a Valentine's text message from an admirer, a fit, handsome, abled-bodied rugby player she had previously dated and who was known to Pistorius, but this was not clarified. He also knew that Reeva had met a former fiancé for coffee, someone with whom she had been in a relationship for five years, the day before she died. It also became clear during the trial that Pistorius phoned her four times in twenty minutes during that meeting. From the evidence, Pistorius also spent an hour on the phone to his ex-girl-friend on his way home earlier that same evening and may well have been sending messages himself, which may have upset Reeva. However, she was not the sort of woman who would have tolerated his infidelity, unlike previous girlfriends on whom he had cheated.

Something she discussed with her close friends shortly before she died was that, just as her career was about to take off, she was also asked by Pistorius to accompany him on his world travels to sporting events, putting her career on hold. This became an issue within the relationship.

EAR-WITNESSES

During the trial, neighbours submitted evidence to the court about a fight they heard that started at least two hours before Pistorius used his firearm to shoot and kill Reeva, at 3.15 a.m. He claimed they were in bed sleeping at around 10.30 p.m. Two other witnesses who lived diago-nally across the road from the athlete were woken up two hours before the shooting to the sounds of a woman's voice raised in argument. This was all contested by Pistorius's defence, casting doubt on the evidence: first they queried the order of events that morning and then they called an expert witness who specializes in how sound travels and questioned what could have been heard by the neighbours, given the distance they lived from the house.

All three of the witnesses were professional people who held respon-sible positions in life and did not know the athlete or Reeva. The main witness was a lecturer at the local university. She described to the court how she was wrenched from her sleep by the distinct blood-curdling screams of a woman in desperate distress, which wafted across the open stands and through the wide-open windows of her house, which was 177 metres away from the crime scene. The screams were soon snuffed out by what the witness described as the distinctive crack of four gunshots. As the shots came to an end, so did the woman's screams. The neigh-bours only offered their story when they heard Oscar Pistorius's claim, in his bail application, that he had mistaken Reeva for an intruder. The witnesses' evidence suggested that, crucially, there were screams *before* the gunshots were fired. The husband of the main witness also confirmed that he too was woken up by a woman's screams.

The pathologist's evidence proved that the food found in Reeva's stomach at the post-mortem was consumed no more than two hours prior to her death around 3.15 a.m., which put her up and awake at 1 a.m. This was contrary to Pistorius's contention that the couple were in bed sleeping after 10 p.m. Another witness, a doctor, heard repeated screams from a woman who sounded as if she was in severe emotional anguish, 'almost scared out of her mind'. Like the other two neighbours, all three were adamant, under cross-examination, that the person screaming hysterically was a woman.

As the estate where Pistorius lived was renowned for having state of the art security, it had no history of crime, let alone violent home invasions. It was also odd that Pistorius's two guard dogs did not alert him to a possible intruder on the night that he shot Reeva.

Whoever Pistorius thought was behind the door, firing at such close range meant that when he finished there would be a body on that bathroom floor. Even though the state was charging Pistorius with the murder of Reeva from multiple gunshot wounds, he was also charged with three other firearms-related offences. And although Pistorius said to the first witnesses on the scene that he thought Reeva was an intruder, it was the case that he shot with the clear intention to kill. An error in persona does not affect the intention to kill a human being. In the trial the state failed to prove murder because it accepted Pistorius's version that he lacked intent in that he genuinely believed that it was an intruder in the toilet.

A VOICE FROM THE GRAVE

Here is just one of Reeva's Whatsapp messages to Pistorius during their short relationship, many of which were read out in full during the trial. They can help us to understand some of his envious behaviour from early on in the relationship.

You are always picking on me – you do everything to throw tantrums in front of me, to put me down … I am scared of you sometimes and how you snap at me for no reason in front of people. I get snapped at … stop chewing gum, do this, don't do that …

In her own words, Reeva said at times in her long messages to him that she was scared of him; she describes his jealousy and temper, and hinted at an abusive relationship. It was the instances of apparent fear and belittlement that the prosecution in the trial believed characterized the relationship. The defence in the trial argued that most of the other messages between the two were loving and only 10 per cent were fearful. Does that mean, then, the prosecution argued, that only 10 per cent of your body has cancer!

Pistorius suffered from the type of envy that results in action, which is a mental disorder as it contains so much murderous rage, even though envy is not considered a psychiatric disorder. He was not psychiatrically impaired and he did know right from wrong the night he shot Reeva. But it was a disaster just waiting to happen. it is important to point out that with such an unstable psychic foundation due to his traumatic experiences as an infant, his is a disturbance that is also based on shame and deprivation going back a long way to when he had a traumatic operation at eleven months old, at a pre-verbal stage of his development.

When Pistorius, a skilled user of firearms, was cross-examined by the prosecution, he was asked to confirm that he fired four shots into the door of the toilet knowing that he would kill the person on the other side of the door. His reply was that if he wanted to kill the person, he would have fired higher! Chillingly, by firing lower, even if he had not killed Reeva, he certainly would have blown her legs to pieces, rendering her just as disabled as he is.

On another occasion, Pistorius was with a group of friends in a crowded restaurant one lunchtime. He fired a shot under the table and the bullet grazed the foot of a friend he was sitting with. He denied firing the gun and the friend took the blame, explaining that Pistorius did not want the publicity as it would affect his relationship with his sponsors.

He was later found guilty of discharging a firearm in a public place during his trial.

Reeva's mother has also written a book and in it she says, 'Her clothes were packed. There is no doubt in our minds: she had decided to leave Oscar that night.' Reeva was very vocal about crimes against women and her mother is convinced that she would never have remained silent if her life was in danger – as it was.[7]

Pistorius may well have shot Reeva to prevent her from ruining his 'squeaky clean' public image by using her mobile, when she had locked herself in the toilet, possibly to call the police, or to alert somebody to the fact that he was armed and, based on her screams, her life was in danger.

Although Pistorius was acquitted of premeditated murder, before sentencing, in the summing-up, the prosecutor ended his five-day cross-examination with a stark summary of what he believed happened: 'You fired four shots through the door whilst knowing she was standing behind that door ... She was locked into the bathroom and you armed yourself with the sole purpose of shooting and killing her.'

We know that there were only two people present: Reeva, who was dead, and Pistorius, who had admitted shooting her and who now, by his own admission, was trying to save his own life. Whatever happened before the shooting, Pistorius may have feared his entire professional future would be affected by the publicity should Reeva live to tell the tale.

The first detective at the scene of the crime arrived shortly after the shooting. A policeman for twenty-five years, he said that in his experience it was an open and shut case of deliberate murder after a raging lovers' argument. Reading his evidence at the bail hearing, he stated that Reeva Steenkamp was still wearing the clothes she had arrived in the previous day, not her nightwear. Her bag was packed to go, on the sofa in the bedroom, including her toiletries. This was around 4.30 a.m., when he was called to investigate and found her dead body at the foot of the stairs, where the athlete had carried her, while he waited for an ambulance. Reeva was pronounced dead by the paramedics. Pistorius was eventually arrested and taken to the police station, where he was charged with her murder.

Currently, at the time of writing, the state will appeal against the sentence, claiming that the judge made an error of law by not convicting him of *dolus eventualis* – indirect intent – a type of murder charge used when a person realizes there is a possibility that their actions might kill someone but carries on regardless.

As I have already made clear, there is a difference between jealousy and envy. One could tolerate and survive being on the receiving end of jealous behaviour, but one could not necessarily survive an envious attack with murderous intent, which I believe was the case in this double tragedy. The lives to two gifted young people were shattered.

CONCLUDING REMARKS

Oscar Pistorius's background has played a major part in determining his insecurities and history of difficulties during relationships. Because of his early childhood history, he did not mature. Faced with his own emptiness, he tried to destroy the happiness of others around him, not being able to bear to see freedom and confidence in the women with whom he had relationships. He suffered deep-rooted post-traumatic stress disorder as an infant, caused by the discomfort and pain he must have felt as a baby after his legs were amputated. He experienced his parents' divorce when he was seven years old and was abandoned by his father. His mother's neurotic behaviour and paranoia were constant features of his developmental years.

To summarize the facts that emerged during the trial, we learned that Pistorius had a chequered emotional history when it came to relationships, always cheating on his current girlfriend with an ex; that his reckless and irresponsible use of firearms led to three separate charges; that he had a love of powerful cars which he drove dangerously – a fact confirmed by a colleague whom he once drove to the airport; that he had a speedboat accident in 2009 in which he suffered serious injuries and nearly died; that a girlfriend of a woman he dated before he met

Reeva was claiming damages against him because he aggressively slammed a door on her while she was at a party in his house (the injury to her foot required surgery and in January 2013 Pistorius settled out of court).

These things demonstrate an aspect of self-envy. One part of Oscar Pistorius is an Olympic gold medallist, a national hero, as famous in South Africa as Nelson Mandela. But another part is totally self-destructive, sabotaging his success, destroying the brilliant future he could have had. And he takes another young person's life by shooting her in a murderous rage, destroying her future too. All of this can be explained by the fact that he needs to express his disability somehow, through his actions and his behaviour, as a way of articulating his suffering, especially as he was brought up to believe that he did not have a disability and was the same as everyone else.

Pistorius has demonstrated, by his behaviour, a central feature of envious ill will: the determination to undermine happiness and replace contentment and calm with agitation and anger, doubt and despair.

Envy is not innate. We are not all born with it. The underlying dynamics operating in envious individuals are always based on deprivation at an early age, which causes deep resentment and a feeling of injustice. These individuals display unstable and intense emotions and are extremely narcissistic, coupled with having zero degrees of empathy, which means they are unable to feel or appreciate feelings which are not their own (as described in the research of Simon Baron-Cohen). Which means that being in a relationship with an envious person can only be emotional abuse.

CHAPTER 12

OSCAR PISTORIUS: ON REFLECTION

I WAS INITIALLY impressed by the fact that very little had been presented during his trial to argue that Oscar Pistorius was 'not in his right mind' at the time of the shooting; or even that this was a case of 'diminished responsibility', a term used in the UK in order for an offender to serve their sentence in a special hospital. I am sure that if Pistorius had been diagnosed as having a psychiatric illness at the time, he would have avoided prison and served his sentence in a special hospital. No doubt it would also have seriously affected his sponsorship with Nike and the five other brands from which he was earning a considerable amount of money at the time of the shooting.

All we really know was that Oscar Pistorius claimed he made a mistake in believing that there was an intruder in his house. This was his story and he was sticking to it. He also underwent a month's psychiatric evaluation before sentencing, only for the court to be told that he was of sane mind when he fired four shots, through the toilet door, and that he knew right from wrong.

A diagnosis of Global Anxiety Disorder (GAD), which was presented to the court by a forensic psychiatrist two weeks before sentencing, prompted the judge to send Pistorius for a psychiatric evaluation, as she claimed that the court was not experienced in understanding this level of expertise and terminology. If the judge had not taken that action, which irritated Pistorius's defence team at the time, it could later have been argued that Pistorius was not given a fair trial. The GAD theory was soon dismissed by the psychiatrists evaluating him during the month that he attended a psychiatric hospital prior to sentencing.

In presenting a diagnosis of GAD, the forensic psychiatrist explained to the court that Pistorius's fight or flight response (common in all humans and animals when sensing a danger to their lives) would have been to fight, not flee, or freeze, due to his limited mobility when not wearing his prosthetic legs. The judge gave him the benefit of the doubt by asking further experts to confirm that this could have been a determining factor in the explanation of Pistorius's actions at the time of the shooting.

It seems that this evaluation was an attempt by Pistorius's defence to get him off the charge of murder. Perhaps then he would be acquitted and retain his reputation and continue in his professional career as an athlete. After all, Pistorius had hired the best legal brains money could buy.

Everybody has probably experienced envy at one time or another. Owing to its confusional characteristics, envy is always subtly disguised and never appears in a straightforward manner, as this awful tragedy shows. Also, the availability of guns to delusional persons is especially problematic.

Oscar Pistorius is eligible for release into house arrest after just ten months in prison. He was due to be free in August 2015, but this has been disputed. The sentence had given Reeva Steenkamp's parents 'a sort of closure', but, as her mother said, there would be no final closure without Reeva, 'unless you can magic her back'.

Pistorius will not be allowed to return to competitive sport until his sentence officially terminates in 2019. There is nothing left of the icon he had once been, one of the most celebrated athletes in the world.*

---

* At the time of writing, Oscar Pistorius has now had his verdict upgraded from culpable homicide to murder which carries a fifteen year sentence. Five supreme court of appeal judges dismissed Pistorius's evidence as "vacillating and untruthful".

Finally, to recapitulate, using the hypothesis of forensic psychotherapy, this case is an example of how the actual behavioural details of a crime become crucial as a means to *understand* better the psychological profile and disturbance of the offender in relation to his offending behaviour. These individuals are unique in that they *demonstrate* what is going on in their minds by the behaviour they act out. In the case of Oscar Pistorius, the model used in forensic psychotherapy, I believe, places particular emphasis upon the developmental importance of the experiences he had in his early maturational years. His early developmental misfortunes are predicted to have had a significant effect on his adult behaviour. His unresolved anger and resentment, coupled with confusion about who he was, did explode, like a bomb, at a time in his life when a crisis caused his self-reliance to break down, leading him to lose control and kill.

CONCLUSION: ENVY IS NOT INNATE

CONSIDERABLE CONTROVERSY STILL exists to this day among psychoanalysts about whether envy is a primary aggressive impulse or not. Although a majority think that envy is a later derivative of character traits, interests and attitudes which only achieve their permanent status towards the end of psychosexual development, others see it as a secondary force which may have positive and adaptive consequences for ongoing development, or may lead to malignant psychopathology.[1] Both viewpoints treat envy as a purely reactive event.

However, centuries of religious thought, philosophical analysis, historical inquiry and literary imagination suggest that envy is a sort of sickness. There is also empirical evidence for the claims that envy causes poor health in the form of real effects on mental and physical well-being.[2]

Having spent many years researching, among other things, the topic of envy, I can say that, in my experience, envy does not appear by itself. We are not born with it, as the psychoanalytical literature still soldiers on steadfastly believing. I disagree profoundly with that view. I can also say that envy is not an eternal and unavoidable quality of an individual. It develops from an atmosphere of insecurity, born out of serious deprivation in the younger developmental years. These developmental misfortunes render an individual severely disturbed when it comes to relationships in later life. In this respect, envy is a *secondary phenomenon*, not an innate disposition we are all born with. Therefore, envy can be regarded as a drawback or flaw which affects the individual's entire life, as well as those to whom he is attached or with whom he has an intimate relationship. That is why the concept of envy has entered the field of philosophical thinking.[3]

By just accepting that envy is one of the seven deadly sins, and assuming that it is inborn, we fail as an intellectual community. We tend to avoid important fundamental questions rather than finding ways to engage with them so as to advance our understanding of the darker side of human nature.

It is important to recognize that many emotional disturbances are the legacy of another's inhumanity.[4] Infants do not create depriving, abusive and neglectful parents, but are found in substantial numbers suffering from this trauma before going on to adult life with personality damage, which manifests itself in difficulties in relationships.

I have always considered the psychoanalytical theory of constitutional envy to be its greatest weakness. To look beyond the brick wall of a doctrine that is held up to be a universal explanation for human ills and at the same time obscures the part played by unsatisfactory life experiences has led me to formulate a different account of early mental processes. Having a model of mental health is an extremely important benchmark to differentiate it from mental illness, as we can see in the examples I have given here.

I believe that the nature of instinct is to enhance the chances of survival. Therefore, to believe that we are all born with a death wish is a biological absurdity. A baby is born sane and with a desire for life. If all goes well, the baby will develop a healthy relationship and establish itself in a dependent interaction with a caring other. This is the vital concept.

The tendency to feel a pang of envy at another's good fortune is universal. Usually, the feeling is fleeting. It is not a spur to action, or even a source of lasting unhappiness. When it is, it has crossed the border between the normal and the pathological. In such cases, envy is not a preference, it is a disease.

Envy is a complex phenomenon requiring much more research and much greater understanding; it cannot simply be seen as an explanation for attacks on good experiences. In clinical forensic practice, it is relatively common to come across a level of destructiveness and murderousness that is of such intensity that it could be interpreted as resembling an anti-life force in whose powerful grip someone will systematically destroy any hopes, aspirations, good feelings, etc. in himself and others, as was the case with Oscar Pistorius. That is why psychoanalysis can be particularly useful for understanding envy and, in Pistorius's case, the unconscious side of this emotion. It deals mainly with unconscious aspects of our behaviour, making it possible to gain access to the deep subjectivity of the envious person and understand the feelings, ideas and phantasies associated with this complex emotion.

I am aware that when one is immersed in studying a subject there is a tendency to see it everywhere. This can be due to an acute sensitivity to its presence, however disguised. Envy is one of the most painful emotions: people are ashamed of it and are loath to admit to it. But envy is as old as humanity, and until we understand the problems it creates for us, we cannot deal with them. I hope that this book will prove helpful in unravelling a very complex and complicated form of mental disorder that we may all encounter, at one time or another, in everyday life.

I will end with a quote from the French-Swiss doctor and psychologist Paul Tournier, who shies away from the problem of envy and discusses instead the guilt of being unequal, the pain of comparing ourselves with others and how we play down our qualities in order not to be envied:

But in all fields, even those of culture and art, other people's judgement exercises a paralysing effect. Fear of criticism kills spontaneity; it prevents men from expressing themselves freely, as they are. Much courage is needed to paint a picture, to write a book, to erect a building designed along new architectural lines, or to formulate an independent opinion or an original idea. Any new concept, any creation falls foul of a host of critics. Those who criticize most are the ones who create nothing. But they form a powerful wall which we all fear to run into more than we admit.[5]

NOTES

INTRODUCTION

1. Melanie Klein, 'Notes on Some Schizoid Mechanisms', in *Envy and Gratitude and Other Works 1946–1963* (London, Hogarth, 1975).

2. Klein, *Envy and Gratitude and Other Works 1946–1963.*

CHAPTER 1: JEALOUSY AND ENVY

1. Jilly Cooper, *Sunday Times*, 25 April 1971, cited in Joseph H. Berke, *The Tyranny of Malice* (London, Summit Books, 1988).

2. Berke, *The Tyranny of Malice*, p. 19.

3. Harry S. Sullivan, *The Interpersonal Theory of Psychiatry* (New York, Norton, 1953), p. 347.

CHAPTER 2: ENVY IS AS OLD AS MANKIND

1. Immanuel Kant, *Metaphysik der Sitten*, 1797, in K. Vorlander (ed.), *Sämtliche Werke*, Vol. 3 (4th edn, Leipzig, Felix Meiner, 1922), p. 316.

2. Arthur Schopenhauer, *Sämtliche Werke*, edited by A. Hubscher, Vol. 6 (Leipzig, 1939), pp. 223–39.

3. Søren Kierkegaard, *Sygdommen til Døden*, 1849 (*The Sickness unto Death*), in H. O. Lange (ed.), *Samlede Vaerker*, Vol. XI (Copenhagen, 1920–30), pp. 197ff.

4. Friedrich Nietzsche, *Collected Works*, Vol. 11 (London, 1910), p. 50.

CHAPTER 3: SHAME AND ENVY

1. See Joseph H. Berke, 'Shame and Envy', in D. L. Nathanson (ed.), *The Many Faces of Shame* (London, Guilford, 1987), p. 32.

2. Patricia Polledri, *Envy is Not Innate: A New Model of Thinking* (London, Karnac, 2012), p. 87.

3. Judith Trowell and Alicia Etchegoyen, *The Importance of Fathers* (London, Brunner-Routledge, 2002), p. 79.

4. Mary Ayers, *Mother–Infant Attachment and Psychoanalysis* (London, Brunner-Routledge, 2003), pp. 64–5.

5. Donald L. Nathanson, *Shame and Pride: Affect, Sex and the Birth of the Self* (New York, W. W. Norton, 1992).

6. See Polledri, *Envy is Not Innate*, p. 96, and James Gilligan, *Violence: Reflections on Our Deadliest Epidemic* (London, Jessica Kingsley, 2000), p. 213.

7. Nathanson, *Shame and Pride*, p 212.

CHAPTER 4: SELF-ENVY

1. Wifred Bion, *Second Thoughts: Selected Papers on Psychoanalysis* (London, William Heinemann, 1967).

2. Warren Colman, 'Envy, Self Esteem and the Fear of Separateness', *British Journal of Psychotherapy*, Vol. 7, No. 4, 1991, p. 365.

CHAPTER 5: ENVY AND PERVERSE BEHAVIOUR

1. See Patrick Gallwey, 'Psychotic and Borderline Processes', in C. Cordess and M. Cox (eds), *Forensic Psychotherapy* (London, Jessica Kingsley, 1996), p. 159.

CHAPTER 6: WOMB ENVY

1. See Catherine B. Silver, 'Womb Envy: Loss and Grief of the Maternal Body', *Psychoanalytic Review*, Vol. 94, No. 3, 2007, p. 411.

2. Karen Horney, 'The Dread of Woman', *International Journal of Psychoanalysis*, Vol. 13, 1932.

3. Adam Jukes, *Why Men Hate Women* (London, Free Association, 1993).

4. Patricia Polledri, 'Envy Revisited', *British Journal of Psychotherapy*, Vol. 20, No. 2, 2003, pp. 195–218.

5. See, for example, D. S. Jaffe, 'The Masculine Envy of Women's Procreative Function', *Journal of American Psychoanalytical Association*, Vol. 16, 1968, pp. 521–48; Jukes, *Why Men Hate Women*; Eva Kittay, 'Mastering Envy: From Freud's Narcissistic Wounds to Bettleheim's Symbolic Wounds to a Vision of Healing', *Psychoanalytic Review*, Vol. 82, No. 1, 1995, pp. 125–58; J. A. Knight,

'Unusual Case: False Pregnancy in a Male', *Medical Aspects of Human Sexuality*, March 1971, pp. 58–67; Rosalind Minsky, '"Too Much of a Good Thing": Control or Containment in Coping with Change', *Psychoanalytic Studies*, Vol. 1, No. 4, 1999, pp. 391–405; Patricia Polledri, *Envy is Not Innate: A New Model of Thinking* (London, Karnac, 2012).

6. Susan Long, *The Perverse Organisation and Its Deadly Sins* (London, Karnac, 2008), p. 93.

7. Luce Irigaray, *Sexes et parentes* (Paris, Minuit, 1987); Jukes, *Why Men Hate Women*; Kittay, 'Mastering Envy'; Rosalind Minsky, 'Reaching Beyond Denial-sight and In-sight, a Way Forward?', *Free Association*, Vol. 35, No. 3, 1995, pp. 326–51.

8. Joseph H. Berke, 'Womb Envy', *Journal of Melanie Klein and Object Relations*, Vol. 15, No. 3, 1997, p. 444.

9. Joseph H. Berke, *The Tyranny of Malice* (London, Summit Books, 1988), p. 101.

10. Otto Kernberg, *Aggression in Personality Disorders and Perversions* (New Haven, CT, Yale University Press, 1992), p. 25.

11. Polledri, 'Envy Revisited'.

12. Berke, *The Tyranny of Malice*, p. 76.

13. Polledri, *Envy is Not Innate*.

CHAPTER 7: ENVY, NARCISSISM AND ZERO DEGREES OF EMPATHY

1. Jon Elster, 'Norms of Revenge', *Ethics*, Vol. 100, No. 4, July 1990, pp. 862–85.

2. See, for example, Simon Baron-Cohen, *Zero Degrees of Empathy* (London, Penguin, 2012); Joseph H. Berke, *The Tyranny of Malice* (London, Summit Books, 1988); Arthur Hyatt Williams, *Cruelty, Violence and Murder* (London, Karnac, 1998).

3. Berke, *The Tyranny of Malice*, p. 71.

4. Ibid.

5. Otto Kernberg, *Borderline Conditions and Pathological Narcissism* (New York, Jason Aronson, 1975).

6. Baron-Cohen, *Zero Degrees of Empathy*, pp. 30ff.

CHAPTER 8: ENVY IN ACADEMIA

1. Glenn Hudak, 'Envy and Goodness in Academia', *Peace Review*, Vol. 12, No. 4, 2000, pp. 607–12.

CHAPTER 10: WHAT IS FORENSIC PSYCHIATRY AND PSYCHOTHERAPY?

1. Patricia Polledri, *Envy is Not Innate: A New Model of Thinking* (London, Karnac, 2012), p. 3.

2. Arthur Hyatt Williams and Christopher Cordess, 'The Criminal Act and Acting Out', in C. Cordess and M. Cox (eds), *Forensic Psychotherapy* (London, Jessica Kingsley, 1996), pp. 14–15.

CHAPTER 11: OSCAR PISTORIUS

1. John Carlin, *Chase Your Shadow: The Trials of Oscar Pistorius* (London, HarperCollins, 2014), p. 71.

2. Ibid.

3. Melinda Ferguson and Patricia Taylor, *Oscar: An Accident Waiting to Happen* (Johannesburg, MF Books, 2014).

4. Ibid.

5. Otto Kernberg, *Aggression in Personality Disorders and Perversions* (New Haven, CT, Yale University Press, 1992).

6. Van der Leek, N., *Recidivist Acts: Oscar Pistorius and the Crime That Shocked the World* (e-book, 2014).

7. June Steenkamp, *Reeva: A Mother's Story* (London, Little, Brown, 2014) and interview on GMTV after publication of book.

CONCLUSION

1. W. G. Joffe, 'A Critical Review of the Status of the Envy Concept', *International Journal of Psycho-Analysis*, Vol. 50, No. 4, 1969, pp. 537–44.

2. Richard H. Smith, *Envy: Theory and Research* (London, Oxford University Press, 2008), Chapter 16.

3. Patricia Polledri, *Envy is Not Innate: A New Model of Thinking* (London, Karnac, 2012).

4. Geoffrey Fisk, 'Envy and the Darkness of Human Nature', *Evangelicals Now*, August 1966.

5. Paul Tournier, *Escape from Loneliness* (Philadelphia, Westminster Press, 1962), p. 98.

FURTHER READING

Ayers, M., *Mother–Infant Attachment and Psychoanalysis* (London, Brunner-Routledge, 2003)

Baron-Cohen, S., *Zero Degrees of Empathy* (London, Penguin, 2012)

Beckelman, L., *Envy* (USA, Silver Burdett Press, 1995)

Berke, J., 'Womb Envy', *Journal of Melanie Klein and Object Relations*, Vol. 15, No. 3, 1997, pp. 443–4

Berke, J. H., *The Tyranny of Malice* (London, Summit Books, 1988)

Berke, J. H., *Why I Hate You and You Hate Me: The Interplay of Envy, Greed, Jealousy and Narcissism in Everyday Life* (London, Karnac, 2012)

Berke, J. H., 'Shame and Envy', in D. L. Nathanson (ed.), *The Many Faces of Shame* (London, Guilford, 1987)

Bion, W., *Second Thoughts: Selected Papers on Psychoanalysis* (London, William Heinemann, 1967)

Bion, W., 'Attacks on Linking', *International Journal of Psychoanalysis*, Vol. 40, 1959, pp. 306–10

Burrows, K., *Ideas in Psychoanalysis: Envy* (London, Icon Books, 2002)

Carlin, J., *Chase Your Shadow: The Trials of Oscar Pistorius* (London, HarperCollins, 2014)

Cleckley, H. M., *The Mask of Sanity* (rev. edn, New York, Plume, 1982)

Colman, W., 'Envy, Self Esteem and the Fear of Separateness', *British Journal of Psychotherapy*, Vol. 7, No. 4, 1991, pp. 356–67

Diagnostic and Statistical Manual of Mental Disorders (4th edn, text revision (DSM-1V-TR), American Psychiatric Association, 2000)

Elster, J., 'Norms of Revenge', *Ethics*, Vol. 100, No. 4, July 1990, pp. 862–85

Epstein, J., *Envy: The Seven Deadly Sins* (Oxford and New York, Oxford University Press, 2003)

Ferguson, M., and Taylor, P., *Oscar: An Accident Waiting to Happen* (Johannesburg, MF Books, e-book, 2014)

Fisk, G., 'Envy and the Darkness of Human Nature', *Evangelicals Now*, August 1966

Foster, G., *Tzintkuntzan: Mexican Peasants in a Changing World* (Boston, Little, Brown, 1965)

Freud, S., *Introductory Lectures on Psycho-Analysis*, SE 15, 16 (London, Hogarth Press, 1916–17)

Gallwey, P., 'Psychotic and Borderline Processes', in C. Cordess and M. Cox (eds), *Forensic Psychotherapy* (London, Jessica Kingsley, 1996)

Gerrod Parrot, W., and Smith, R. H., 'Distinguishing the Experiences of Envy and Jealousy', *Journal of Personality and Social Psychology*. Vol. 64, No. 6. 1993, pp. 906–20

Gilligan, J., *Violence: Reflections on Our Deadliest Epidemic* (London, Jessica Kingsley, 2000)

Gilligan, J., 'Exploring Shame in Special Settings', in C. Cordess and M. Cox (eds), *Forensic Psychotherapy* (London, Jessica Kingsley, 1996)

Horney, K., 'The Dread of Woman', *International Journal of Psychoanalysis*, Vol. 13, 1932, pp. 348–60

Hudak, G. H., 'Envy and Goodness in Academia', *Peace Review*, Vol. 12, No. 4, 2000, pp. 607–12

Hyatt Williams, A., *Cruelty, Violence and Murder* (London, Karnac, 1998)

Hyatt Williams, A., and Cordess, C., 'The Criminal Act and Acting Out', in C. Cordess and M. Cox (eds), *Forensic Psychotherapy* (London, Jessica Kingsley, 1996)

Irigaray, L., *Sexes et parentes* (Paris, Minuit, 1987; translated as *Sexes and Genealogies*, New York, Columbia University Press, 1973)

Jaffe, D. S., 'The Masculine Envy of Women's Procreative Function', *Journal of American Psychoanalytical Association*, Vol. 16, 1968, pp. 521–48

Joffe, W. G., 'A Critical Review of the Status of the Envy Concept', *International Journal of Psycho-Analysis*, Vol. 50, No. 4, 1969, pp. 537–44

Joseph, B., 'Envy in Everyday Life', *Psychoanalytic Psychotherapy*, Vol. 2, 1986, pp. 13–22

Jukes, A., *Why Men Hate Women* (London, Free Association, 1993)

Kant, I., *Metaphysik der Sitten*, 1797 (*The Metaphysics of Morals*), in K. Vorlander (ed.), *Sämtliche Werke*, Vol. 3 (4th edn, Leipzig, Felix Meiner, 1922)

Kernberg, O., *Borderline Conditions and Pathological Narcissism* (New York, Jason Aronson, 1975)

Kernberg, O., *Aggression in Personality Disorders and Perversions* (New Haven, CT, Yale University Press, 1992)

Kierkegaard, S., *Sygdommen til Døden*, 1849 (*The Sickness unto Death*), in H. O. Lange (ed.), *Samlede Vaerker*, Vol. XI (Copenhagen, 1920–30)

Kittay, E., 'Mastering Envy: From Freud's Narcissistic Wounds to Bettleheim's Symbolic Wounds to a Vision of Healing', *Psychoanalytic Review*, Vol. 82, No. 1, 1995, pp. 125–58

Klein, M., *Envy and Gratitude and Other Works 1946–1963* (London, Hogarth, 1975)

Knight, J. A., 'Unusual Case: False Pregnancy in a Male', *Medical Aspects of Human Sexuality*, March 1971, pp. 58–67

Long, S., *The Perverse Organisation and Its Deadly Sins* (London, Karnac, 2008)

McElvaine, R. S., *Eve's Seed: Biology, the Sexes and the Course of History* (New York, McGraw Hill, 2000)

Minsky, R., 'Reaching Beyond Denial-sight and In-sight, a Way Forward?', *Free Association*, Vol. 35, No. 3, 1995, pp. 326–51

Minsky, R., '"Too Much of a Good Thing": Control or Containment in Coping with Change', *Psychoanalytic Studies*, Vol. 1, No. 4, 1999, pp. 391–405

Mollon, P., *Shame and Jealousy: The Hidden Turmoils* (London, Karnac, 2002)

Nathanson, D. L., *Shame and Pride: Affect, Sex and the Birth of the Self* (New York, W. W. Norton, 1992)

Nietzsche, F., *Collected Works*, Vol. 11 (London, 1910)

Pistorius, O., *Blade Runner* (London, Virgin Books, 2009)

Polledri, P., *Envy is Not Innate: A New Model of Thinking* (London, Karnac, 2012)

Polledri, P., 'Munchausen Syndrome by Proxy and Perversion of the Maternal Instinct', *Journal of Forensic Psychiatry*, Vol. 7, No. 3, 1996, pp. 561–2

Polledri, P., 'Forensic Psychotherapy with a Potential Serial Killer', *British Journal of Psychotherapy*, Vol. 13, No. 4, 1997, pp. 473–88

Polledri, P., 'Envy Revisited', *British Journal of Psychotherapy*, Vol. 20, No. 2, 2003, pp. 195–218

Polledri, P., 'Which Version of Perversion Is Womb Envy?', paper read at the 21st International Association of Forensic Psychotherapy Conference, Venice, March 2012

Rycroft, C., *A Critical Dictionary of Psychoanalysis* (Harmondsworth, Penguin, 1968)

Salovey, P., *The Psychology of Jealousy and Envy* (New York, Guilford Press, 1991)

Salovey, P., and Rodin, J., 'Jealousy and Envy: The Dark Side of Emotion', *Psychology Today*, February 1985, pp. 32–4

Schoeck, H., *Envy: A Theory of Social Behaviour* (Indianapolis, Liberty Fund, 1987; first published in German, 1966)

Schopenhauer, A., *Sämtliche Werke*, edited by A. Hubscher, Vol. 6 (Leipzig, 1939)

Shimmel, S., 'Envy in Jewish Literature and Thought', in R. H. Smith (ed.), *Envy: Theory and Research* (London, Oxford University Press, 2008), pp. 17–38

Silver, C. B., 'Womb Envy: Loss and Grief of the Maternal Body', *Psychoanalytic Review*, Vol. 94, No. 3, 2007, pp. 409–30

Smith, R. H., *Envy: Theory and Research* (London, Oxford University Press, 2008)

Steenkamp, J., *Reeva: A Mother's Story* (London, Little, Brown, 2014)

Stoller, R. J., *Perversion: The Erotic Form of Hatred* (New York, Pantheon Books, 1975)

Sullivan, H. S., *The Interpersonal Theory of Psychiatry* (New York, Norton, 1953)

Tournier, P., *Escape from Loneliness* (Philadelphia, Westminster Press, 1962)

Trowell, J., and Etchegoyen, A., *The Importance of Fathers* (London, Brunner-Routledge, 2002)

Van der Leek, N., *Recidivist Acts: Oscar Pistorius and the Crime That Shocked the World* (e-book, 2014)

Wiener, M., and Bateman, B., *Behind the Door: The Oscar Pistorius and Reeva Steenkamp Story* (South Africa, Pan Macmillan, 2014)

Winnicot, Donald, *Playing and Reality* (London, Tavistock, 1971)

Winnicott, Donald, *Deprivation and Delinquency* (London, Tavistock, 1984)

Zhang, X., and Sang, Y., *Chinese Lives* (New York, Pantheon, 1987)